I0814189

Creating Safe, Healthy, and Inclusive Schools

CREATING SAFE, HEALTHY, AND INCLUSIVE SCHOOLS

Challenges and Solutions

EDITED BY
Christopher C. Morphew,
Vanya C. Jones, *and* Ashley E. Cureton

FOREWORD BY
Michele Gay

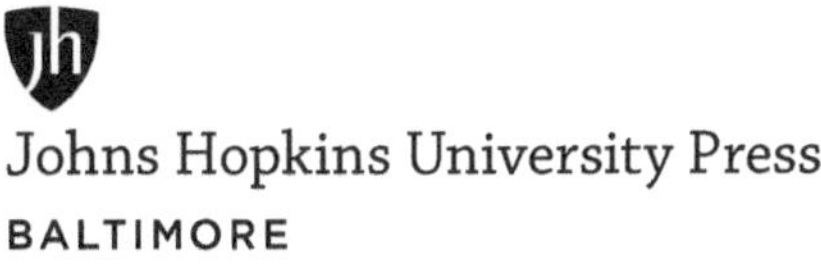

Johns Hopkins University Press
BALTIMORE

Printed in the United States of America on acid-free paper
9 8 7 6 5 4 3 2 1

Johns Hopkins University Press
2715 North Charles Street
Baltimore, Maryland 21218
www.press.jhu.edu

Library of Congress Cataloging-in-Publication Data is available.

A catalog record for this book is available from the British Library.

ISBN 978-1-4214-4978-4 (hardcover)
ISBN 978-1-4214-4979-1 (ebook)

Contents

Foreword

MICHELE GAY

On a perfectly ordinary December morning in Sandy Hook, Connecticut, I lost my seven-year-old daughter, Josephine. I had made her a special breakfast and cuddled with her on the couch before driving her to school that morning. I had sent her two older sisters to school ahead of her, one to the intermediate school, the other to Sandy Hook Elementary, both in our town of Newtown. Like any other bustling morning, we had packed lunches, argued over what to wear, and barely made it on time to the bus stop.

With each of my daughters safely off to school, I settled on the couch for a quick coffee and breakfast, only to be interrupted by the ringing of the phone. It was an automated call from the superintendent of schools informing me that the Newtown Schools were all in lockdown. There had been a shooting in one of our schools. It was a simple message that would change my life forever.

Years later, I am still grappling with that message and the news that would follow. It seems as impossible today as it did when I heard it that December day. So impossible that I had hoped it was just a terrible mistake, a misunderstanding I could readily get to the bottom of.

Only, it was not.

As the day wore on, my husband and I would learn an unimaginable truth. Our youngest daughter was gone, killed alongside nineteen of her six- and seven-year-old peers and six of our beloved educators. Our lives and our community would never be the same.

"How could this have happened?" It's a question I asked myself that day and every day since. "These were good schools. Safe schools."

When we chose to move our young family to the Northeast, I had carefully searched for a tight-knit community with low crime, strong schools, and good neighbors. Newtown, Connecticut, checked all the boxes. The school test scores were high, the parents were involved, and they even had a locked, "buzz-in" entry system. "Safety" was a priority. The school conducted regular fire, evacuation, and lockdown drills, and hosted first responders to build relationships and confidence with students. Each of my daughters thrived in the environment—until December 14, 2012.

That day would alter the course of our lives and require us to face a future we never wanted. A future without Josephine. It would be the beginning of a long journey for our family, and for me.

Haunted by these questions, I have committed my life to finding answers. After all, if our school was not safe, how could any school be safe? But what makes a school safe? If you ask ten people, you'll get ten different answers: More security, more school counselors, more technology, more school resource officers, more training, more money . . . the list goes on.

Leaning into my background as an educator, I sought to learn from every expert, approach, and perspective I could find. I attended federal, state, and local leadership meetings and participated in training, from active shooter to restorative practice. And I learned an important truth: there would be no quick fix, no sweeping legislative victory, and no one person, program, or solution that could resolve the complex challenges directly impacting our youngest and most vulnerable citizens as they learn in the most sacred of places—our schools.

If there is one single "answer," it is this: Ensuring the safety of our schools takes all of us, doing the hard work, committed for the long haul, focusing on prevention, preparing for response, and planning for recovery. It is the strategic, intentional, and steady work of parents, students, educators, school-based mental health specialists, school resource officers, public safety professionals, and the community. It takes all of these heroes working *together.*

Out of the ashes of what had been our family of five came something new: the desire and determination to carry on the love and the life of our daughter; to keep her with us; and to make her proud of us. Through her and the support of these heroes, our friends, family, and faith, we carry on.

We have built a legacy in Josephine's honor. A legacy to protect every school and every child, every day. A legacy that has become the mission of *Safe and Sound Schools*, a nonprofit organization established in 2013 to develop a *comprehensive approach* to school safety. One that would bring together all members of the community behind a common goal of ensuring safe school communities for every child, in every school, every day. Ours is an approach that requires all disciplines, all perspectives, all hearts, all minds, and all hands working together to achieve our mission.

It would be perfectly understandable, perhaps even expected, for our focus to fall squarely and narrowly on school violence prevention; but my experience as an educator, a parent, and now an advocate has led me to dig deeper. It has become clear to me that "school safety" is much more than drills, door locks, and violence prevention. The scope of school safety goes far beyond the walls of our schools, extending deeply into our community, where culture and climate begin and basic needs like health and well-being must be met to ensure equal access to learning and achievement during the school day.

Identifying best practices and partners, like behavioral threat assessment and management, bully prevention, school counselors, school resource officers, and evidence-based approaches and programs, like multi-tiered systems of support and social and emotional learning curricula, schools will have a blueprint to build upon and a place to start. This means collaboration is imperative. In fact, it is at the core of what we believe in as an organization.

Since the founding of Safe and Sound Schools, I have been joined by national experts, parents, teachers, administrators, fire, police, emergency medical and mental health professionals across the country and internationally—many of whom have contributed to the writing of this book. We have built a national community committed to the safety of our nation's schools. As a direct result of our lived and learned experiences, Safe and Sound Schools has identified six domains that comprise this collaborative approach, a Framework for Comprehensive School Safety Planning and Development. Those domains include (1) mental and behavioral health; (2) health and wellness; (3) physical safety and security; (4) culture, climate, and community; (5) leadership, law, and policy; and (6) operations and emergency management. Clearly, it takes each of us working together in partnership to strengthen the needed systems in our schools and communities. No domain stands alone and, notably, several domains focus on issues that might not be traditionally connected with "safety" but are essential to creating safe and healthy environments for our children. Each is intertwined with the intent of meeting the needs of our students, caring for the whole child through a whole community approach.

Today, our mission is more important than ever. In an era where schools face unprecedented challenges, myriad and complex health and safety issues, limited resources, and competing demands from inside and outside of the schoolhouse, school safety requires a broader view and a more expansive approach.

Our schools and our students deserve nothing less.

It is a tall order to be certain. Yet it is more important than ever that we rise to the challenge. We must set aside the dangerous temptation of narrowly focused quick fixes and one-size-fits-all approaches that often fail—and in some cases harm—our schools and our children. This requires leadership at every level in the community, not just the schools.

I invite you, as a reader and leader in your school community, to read the chapters of this book with a fresh perspective and renewed commitment to the safety and well-being of our students and school communities. It is up to each of us to work together to build safe school communities where children and youths can learn, grow, and live up to their full potential.

Together we can make a difference. Together, we can make our schools safe and sound.

Michele Gay is a mother, former teacher, and one of the founders of Safe and Sound Schools. After losing her daughter Josephine Grace on December 14, 2012, she chose to act as an advocate for improved safety in our nation's schools.

Acknowledgments

We have been lucky to have the support of many wonderful people to produce this book. It was truly a collective effort. We would like to acknowledge the extraordinary writers who submitted chapters to this book: Michele Gay, Jonathan M. Links, Richard Lofton Jr., Sheldon "Shelly" Greenberg, Odis Johnson Jr., Beth Marshall, Terrinieka W. Powell, Asari Offiong, Holly C. Wilcox, Chris Swanson, Ashley A. Grant, Olivia Marcucci, Douglas J. Mac Iver, Megan Collins, Sara Johnson, Alan Regenberg, Annette Anderson, Andrew Nicklin, and Ruth Faden. Amid the COVID-19 pandemic and other crises plaguing our country, we appreciate your commitment to being a part of this writing project.

We would not have been able to complete this book without the continual support of Taylor Danielle Parnham and Madison Nuzzo. From reading numerous drafts, making edits, and helping us to remain on track as we completed the manuscript, Taylor and Madison were as instrumental to this book getting done as we were. We would like to thank the Johns Hopkins Consortium for School-Based Health Solutions for supporting this project. Thank you so much.

Many thanks to the National Science Foundation, which supported the research for chapter 6 with grant #DRL-1800199. The ideas expressed in this chapter are entirely those of the author.

Thanks also to the funders of the Restorative Practices with Diplomas Now study in chapter 8, which was made possible by a grant from The Atlantic Philanthropies (23220, Evaluation of Restorative Practices, Robert

Balfanz, PI), matching funds from the PepsiCo Foundation, and a grant from the US Department of Education's Office of Innovation and Improvement (U396B100257; Evaluation Extension, Validating the Talent Development–Diplomas Now Secondary School Turnaround Model, Robert Balfanz, PI). The views expressed in this chapter are those of the authors.

The authors of chapter 9 gratefully acknowledge the research contributions of Kelly Beharry, Azka Tariq, Medha Kallem, Akansh Hans, Alice Liu, Madison Wahl, Emily Faxon, Tiana Sepaphour, Matthew Crane, and Rachel Gur-Arie.

Thanks to everyone from Hopkins Press who helped bring this book to fruition. Special thanks to ever-patient editorial director Greg Britton and his incredible team for guiding us through the process of writing this book from its inception to completion.

We are indebted to the young people, school partners, and community leaders who shared their narratives and challenges in building safe schools and learning environments. Their experiences include navigating ongoing and persistent racism and discrimination, underfunding, and restricted resources. We also want to remember the young people who have lost their lives in school shootings and other acts of violence within school and community spaces. We hope that this book sparks a renewed commitment on how to make schools a safer and more equitable environment for *all* children and youths.

Part I

REFRAMING SCHOOL SAFETY AS SAFE AND HEALTHY SCHOOLS

1

(Re)Defining What Constitutes a Safe and Healthy School

CHRISTOPHER C. MORPHEW, PHD, AND JONATHAN M. LINKS, PHD

What Is a Safe School?

What does it mean to call a school "safe"? The answer to this question is neither simple nor clear. Getting closer to an answer reveals important differences among (1) our schools and communities, (2) the role schools play for students and their families, and (3) attitudes and expectations about schools and their function. These differences are the result of policy inequities and the very different roles schools play across diverse communities.

Prior to the COVID-19 pandemic, many policymakers—and the federal government, historically—would define a safe school by a lack of physical violence and crime. In fact, some scholars would claim that schools should be free of all violence. Incidents of violence in our schools—particularly shootings—have inflicted a general trauma and captured the attention of families and policymakers, as Michele Gay notes in the foreword to this book. It is understandable that these events, even if rare, have come to equate a quest for safe schools as "school safety" for millions of Americans and even the Department of Education's National Center on Safe Supportive Learning Environments. From this perspective, a safe school is one that is protective and difficult to enter without permission—with security guards and cameras, for example—and focuses on violence and crime prevention within its fortified walls. This is reasonable: we send our children to school every morning and expect them to come home safely. However, this is a very limited view of a safe school.

This book brings together a set of researchers who study children, schools, equity, social justice, mental health, and school security to demonstrate that "safety" and "safe" are two very different concepts. A focus on safety, for example, necessitates actions that secure schools, includes police (euphemistically referred to as "school resource officers," or SROs), and seeks to reduce violent actions. Improving safety means limiting violent outcomes. Alternately, a focus on safe schools is foundational; it requires addressing the reasons—proactively, if possible—why students and their families might not feel safe in their schools. Safe schools are healthy schools where mental health is promoted and protected, and schools and school leaders adopt a holistic approach to their students' academic, social, and emotional development. That is, safe schools are those that are free from every sort of risk a student might experience, not just violence.

For many students and their families, feeling safe requires that they trust a teacher or administrator with whom they interact, they have school friends, and are free from routine classmate-based trauma, such as bullying. For some students, school may be a sanctuary from an unstable or violent home life or community. School hours may be the only time these students can feel unthreatened—physically, emotionally, or spiritually.

The Organization of This Book

This book is organized into two sections. Part I, Reframing School Safety as Safe and Healthy Schools, includes five chapters authored by early childhood, public health, education, and equity researchers who describe how their work can help us understand what a safe and healthy learning environment means to children and adolescents, and why our focus should be on "safe" rather than "safety." We make this distinction not because school safety isn't important but because the data make clear that challenges related to providing safe and healthy learning environments are far more ubiquitous.

Chapters 2 through 5 provide diverse and empirical evidence-based perspectives that demonstrate how defining a safe and healthy school requires an examination of the educational setting and group. To understand what it means for a student to feel safe and develop in a healthy manner in any setting, educational or otherwise, requires a focus on the environmental conditions that lead to violence, social control, and significant mental health problems. The authors of these chapters highlight the considerations and needs from diverse perspectives for safe schools. In the case of early childhood education, as described by Chris Swanson in chapter 2, creating a safe and developmentally healthy environment requires a focus on pedagogy, training, and facilities. In chapter 3, Holly Wilcox focuses on the growing importance of addressing mental health for schools, not only because mental health problems are typically first observed in school-age children, but because they are linked to learning outcomes across all grades. Likewise, in chapter 4, Beth Marshall, Terrinieka Powell, and Asari Offiong describe a number of approaches to positive youth development, including trauma-informed approaches—all of which are essential to create safe and productive learning environments. These approaches, along with the suicide prevention interventions outlined by Wilcox, can be effective if structured and timed appropriately. In chapter 5, Richard Lofton notes that Black children attending school in urban environments often experience systematic and consistent trauma on their way to school, on the bus, or after school as they return to their neighborhoods, where violence is the norm rather than the exception.

The first section points out that defining "safe" requires a better and deeper understanding of the data documenting whether schools are providing safe and healthy learning environments. Not only may members of different communities define the concept differently, but students may also have a distinct perspective apart from their parents. Black students may take into consideration unique features relative to their White classmates, and nonbinary students may value other things. The books students read and the concepts they discuss in class may contribute to whether they feel safe (Balingit and Rabinowitz 2021). Parents may be reassured by newer facilities, digital technology, high test scores, and school ranking. For some parents, however, the presence of security cameras, SROs, or clearly defined safety procedures indicate a safe school. Having said that, the presence of armed SROs is not without controversy. For some, the presence of SROs may be normative if you have always attended schools with metal detectors and armed guards; if you have never attended a school that employed SROs, you may find their activities frightening and discriminatory. Post-COVID-19 or natural disaster, feeling safe may require the knowledge that you and your family have shelter and food, as well as an understanding of your school's plan to return to a safe environment with vaccination and testing requirements.

The differences in how we define "safe" in schools are also linked to important differences among communities. Schools are both a part of and an extension of communities, after all. While we all want our children to learn in environments free of violence, individual and shared expectations are shaped by experiences. For example, residents of suburbs experiencing low rates of violent crime may place a particularly high value on schools' response to bullying and peer dynamics, whereas parents in ethically or racially diverse communities may place a premium on finding a school with teachers who share ethnic and/or racial heritage with their children and can support unique experiences for their child to succeed. Commuting is also a part of school safety, including routes to school, modes of transportation (e.g., buses, mass transit, or pedestrian), and supervision during transportation. For example, school buses may serve as an important extension of a safe school in rural America, where more students use them for longer distances. This may be different in cities that rely on municipal buses or walking through neighborhoods with stark evidence of violence, with poorly maintained sidewalks and walkways.

In discussions about safe schools, the word "safety" is often used as a synonym for "safe." The chapters of this book document that this is a mistake. A school can, for example, practice good safety practices and still not be a safe space for its students or families. Locked doors, state-of-the-art security measures, and SROs patrolling the halls may reassure some families, but if those SROs discriminate against Black, immigrant, or nonbinary students and arrest students who defy the dress code or break school rules, these students and others will not feel safe. In fact, it has become elucidated that in some instances, in the quest to improve school safety, schools have been made less safe for students from marginalized groups. This is made clear in chapters 4 and 5 in this book, which discuss the trauma Black students face in Baltimore schools and the impact of carceral methods designed to control students' behavior, respectively. The critical distinction between school safety and a safe school (and, by extension, a healthy school) is a central tenet of this book.

How Do We Measure What Constitutes a Safe School?

Traditionally, the government—federal and state—has published reports on school safety. These reports list rates of violence, including bullying, weapons use, and the percentage of students and teachers who report being afraid of being harmed by others on campus. The National Center for Education Statistics (NCES) and the Bureau of Justice Statistics (BJS), part of the Departments of Education and Justice, respectively, jointly produce the annual "A Report on Indicators of School Crime and Safety" (ISCS), which has been one of the definitive publications on school safety (Irwin et al. 2021). A perusal of the ISCS makes clear how school safety has been defined by the federal government. The most recent, the twenty-fourth, version of this report was published in June 2022 (though it is dated 2021 and includes data through 2020) and includes numerous tables on subjects ranging from "violent deaths and school shootings" to "student perceptions of school safety," to "discipline, safety, and security practices." A reader of ISCS can learn, for example, what percentage of high school students reported using alcohol daily or whether eighth-grade boys or girls were more likely to report being bullied.

What is missing from the ISCS is glaring. The word "gang," for example, is found twelve times in the thirty-one-page 2021 report. "Rape" appears nine times. But the same report mentions "depression" and "anxiety" just once each and fails to include a single mention of "mental health." While the 2021 report does report differences among Black, Hispanic, and White students, it focuses on school fights and hate crimes, not rates of arrest by police officers or SROs. Transgender and nonbinary students are not mentioned in this report except where footnotes identify other relevant surveys, nor are students with individualized education plans (IEPs) or autism spectrum disorders. A reader of this report would come away with the clear impression that none of these variables were important when it comes to measuring school safety. This report makes clear that safety in schools may be defined exclusively by instances of violence.

This failure to measure the many dimensions of what constitutes a safe and healthy school is problematic—incredibly so. When metrics focus exclusively on school safety rather than how educational environments contribute to students and their families feeling safe, we—paradoxically—lose sight of what actually constitutes a safe school. The chapters in this book challenge that focus and advocate for a much broader view of what constitutes a safe school. The authors demonstrate that safe schools represent healthy spaces that allow for and promote children developing knowledge, fundamental skills, and socio-emotional competencies such as critical thinking, problem solving, collaboration, and empathy.

What Is a Healthy School?

The World Health Organization (WHO n.d.) defines "health" in its constitution: "Health is a state of complete physical, mental and social well-being and not merely the absence of disease or infirmity." By analogy, we assert that a healthy school is one in which each student (and teacher and administrator) can experience complete physical, mental, and social well-being.

Too often, as a result of the media and policymakers' focus on horrific tragedies like school shootings, however, we have become fixated on physical safety—that is, not even a focus on a safe school, let alone a safe *and healthy* school. In fact, school violence based on traditional metrics of safety has been on the wane in US schools for several decades. What has increased is students who are negatively impacted by mental health disorders, such as anxiety and depression. In addition, schools have become increasingly unsafe and unhealthy for students from underrepresented backgrounds and those with intellectual disabilities. These students are at disproportionate risk for suspension, expulsion, seclusion, and even arrest. While the ISCS does not focus on high-risk students, other reports have shown that sexual minority youth are experiencing violence in schools more than others (Basile et al. 2020). In some cases, this is—ironically—the direct result of our attempts to improve school safety. This book provides a broad set of evidence and perspectives to document that safe and healthy schools are better defined by their inclusive nature, the support services available to all students, and the presence of a well-trained, trusted set of adults equipped with knowledge regarding the best practices and programs to support students' mental health and perceptions of safety.

The findings and trends portrayed in the ISCS are mixed, but they generally describe schools as relatively low in crime. The past decade has seen decreasing rates of criminal victimization, bullying, and fighting on school campuses. Schools also report fewer instances of crime reported by sworn law enforcement, even as the number of SROs on campus has increased dramatically. There are some negative trends as well: Most notably, the 2020–21 academic year saw the largest number of school shootings (93), including the most with fatalities (43). In comparison, there were twenty-three school shootings in the 2000–01 academic year. There were fewer than twenty crimes against persons or property per ten thousand students, which is a crime rate that compares favorably with the vast majority of urban, rural, and suburban communities in the United States. Overall, it is clear that violence in schools is uncommon.

It is striking and alarming, then, that our schools are increasingly becoming armed fortresses. Even as school violence has declined, states and districts have hired and placed more school resource officers in high schools and even elementary schools. Although more states mandate and districts employ SROs, there is no evidence linking this activity to safer schools, and increasing evidence suggests there is a correlation between their presence and *less safe* schools.

This zeal to place police officers in schools has obvious consequences for the criminalization of behavior that, previously, had resulted in a trip to the principal's office or suspension. As a recent report from the ACLU (American Civil Liberties Union) documents, more than 60 percent of school-based arrests in Florida were for misdemeanors. Disorderly conduct was the second most common offense. Even worse is the disproportionate impact on students from at-risk groups. The same ACLU report notes that

74 percent of females arrested for misdemeanors were Black, even though Black girls made up only 22 percent of Florida's female student population. Black students were not the only group to bear the brunt of inequitable arrest outcomes: students with disabilities were three times more likely than the larger population to be arrested, and Native American and Pacific Islanders were twice as likely to be arrested (Whitaker et al. 2019). When we choose to place police officers in schools, we need to understand that this will result in arrests and disproportionate arrests of the students most in need of support or engagement in less carceral approaches like restorative practices, as Ashley Grant and colleagues discuss in chapter 8. Restorative practices focus on building high-quality relationships that stress a foundation of equity to solve problems and provide a sense of belonging and support (Grant and Mac Iver 2021). A National Institute of Justice (NIJ) report (Frederique 2020) points out that there may be a disconnect between how the public views school safety and the data reported in the ISCS showing that schools have been and continue to be relatively free of violence. The NIJ report notes that most well-known data sources show that crime and violence in schools has declined significantly since the 1990s, when these data began to be reported regularly. An exception to this trend has been multiple-victim, school-associated deaths, which declined from 1994 to 2009 but have been increasing since. While still relatively rare, these events are high profile and traumatic for affected families and our national consciousness (as this book's foreword by Michele Gay eloquently notes). A consequence of the attention paid to these tragic, multiple-victim crimes in schools has been the push to fortify schools with school resource officers and hardened facilities that might repel or thwart these efforts.

Measuring (and Reacting To) School Violence during a Mental Health Crisis

While crime and violence in schools has declined, there is clearly a mental health crisis among adolescents. Reports like the ISCS pay scant attention to this rising tide of mental health issues, which Holly Wilcox chronicles in chapter 3, even though this crisis is manifested in several ways that are being documented. Suicide rates among adolescents have increased by 60 percent between 2007 and 2018 (CDC 2020a), including nearly 50 percent more who report making a suicide plan. One in nine female high school students attempted suicide in 2019, according to the Centers for Disease Control's (CDC's) annual survey of Youth Risk Behaviors (CDC 2020a). More than 36 percent of students surveyed by the CDC for its annual report in 2019 reported experiencing "persistent feelings of sadness of hopelessness," up from 26.1 percent in 2009. This latter statistic includes 46.6 percent of surveyed females (CDC 2020a).

Unfortunately, states and districts have chosen to focus on the data from reports like ISCS rather than the CDC survey results. The inordinate efforts to reduce violent crime in schools has come at a cost, which has substantial implications for students' mental health and equitable outcomes. The buildup of SROs, funded by states in the aftermath of Columbine, Newtown, and Parkland, for example, has resulted in a school system that criminalizes bad behavior and funds SROs instead of funding resources to address a growing mental health epidemic. A 2019 report from the ACLU, using first-time data the Department of Education only recently required of school districts, in 2015–16, documented that nearly 14 million students attend schools with police officers but no counselor, nurse, psychologist, or social worker. Nationally, this means that nearly one-third of students attend school with an exclusive focus on violence prevention rather than mental health; in some states, this figure approaches or exceeds 50 percent of all students (Whitaker et al. 2019; US Department of Education 2010).

While it is increasingly common for districts and schools to employ SROs, what receives less attention are other approaches that focus on community building and addressing the root causes of the mental health crisis. While there is no conceptual reason or empirical evidence to suggest that SROs will address the swelling number of students experiencing anxiety or depression, there is a growing body of evidence from education, medicine, public health, and public policy that there are useful strategies that are polar opposites from carceral approaches that focus on punishment, exclusion, and policing.

How the Book's Chapters Extend What We Know about Making Schools Safer and Healthier

The second part of this book—Approaches for Safe and Healthy Schools, which encompasses chapters 6 through 9—provides a critical set of insights and strategies that school leaders and policymakers can employ to improve schools. For example, Sheldon Greenberg's critical discussion of SROs in chapter 7 proposes a number of improvements that can be made to the training, assessment, and practices of SROs—potentially blunting some of the negative impacts that Johnson identifies. Approaches focused on giving students and their school communities problem-solving tools can be effective without a reliance on SROs, as Ashley Grant, Olivia Marcucci, and Douglas Mac Iver outline in chapter 8. They describe how strategies such as restorative practices can teach students and their families communication tactics that result in fewer conflicts and give students developmentally appropriate problem-solving skills. Finally, Megan Collins and the six coauthors of chapter 9 highlight what we have learned from the COVID-19 pandemic about the central role schools play in keeping students safe and healthy and what schools can do now and in the future to improve their focus on children's well-being.

The book's final chapters document that we know less than we should about what constitutes a safe and healthy school because the data we gather, the approaches we assume effective, and the policies we fund in K–12 schools are not designed to improve the number of students and families who feel safe or address the most likely causes of unhealthiness—mental health issues (that arise both organically and as the result of the physical and social environments in which students and their families reside). We gather data on school violence, employ growing numbers of police officers (SROs), and harden the entrances to our schools. However, as Odis Johnson notes in chapter 6, if a community has been traumatized by police action, armed officers in your school and classrooms are simply further reminders of the carceral state and are unlikely to create a perception of safety or protection. Too often, SROs and hardening schools are the focus of resources even as the number of adolescents reporting mental health concerns is growing rapidly and in the face of no evidence that suggests that police officers stop crime in schools. In fact, it is known that SROs—chosen and evaluated without any attention to their knowledge about schools or schoolchildren—do not act without bias, and Black, Brown, or Latinx children are more likely to be arrested, just as students with IEPs and learning disabilities. This is not a recipe for making schools universally safer and healthier places.

In the pursuit to measure violence, eliminate it, and equate the lack of violence with being safe, there is the need for investment and more work. Policymakers and school leaders have failed to recognize that *safety* and *safe* are two different things and not always correlated, and that *safety* and *healthy* are even less connected. In short, it is clear that the traditional approach to improving school safety has not worked. Just as importantly, it has not made schools safe places for marginalized students and ignored the growing mental health crisis. Future efforts must evolve from a focus on safety to making schools safe and healthy places for *all* students. This is essential if we are to improve schools and student learning. Doing so will require us to move beyond issues of safety and examine what is happening in our school communities and prioritizing approaches that address the real challenges that students and teachers face every day. These challenges include violence, but more often they are connected with mental health, issues of trust and equity, and the fallout from the negative impact of the school-to-prison pipeline that has been amplified by contemporary approaches to issues of safety.

Our goal in this book is to address this gap between what policymakers, school leaders, academics, and practitioners know and what we must and should know about creating and maintaining safe and healthy schools. We made the intentional choice to seek out researchers and practitioners from education, public health, and medicine who spend time in schools and in their research figuring out what produces schools where students feel supported and trusted, where parents are given tools to understand and engage in their children's development, and where teachers, school staff, and administrators believe mental health is an essential ingredient to high-quality schools. Readers will learn about diverse strategies and evidence-based research that reframes how we can think about schools so that the focus can move from *safety* to *safe and healthy*, which is a more efficacious and comprehensive way of thinking about how we can make school communities welcoming, supportive, and trusted spaces for all. In this regard, integral to becoming a safe and healthy school is providing school-based strategies for teachers and students. Restorative practices and other evidenced-based practices provide an opportunity to teach students democratic skills that can help them constructively communicate when they feel unsafe or that others have destroyed trust. This contrasts with approaches like hardening schools and employing (largely untrained) police officers who do not teach students anything about how they can contribute to their own development and health, and instead reinforce the idea that some communities and their residents require carceral approaches to social control. Ultimately, this book represents an evidence-based plea to radically revise our entire conceptualization and approach to school safety, ushering in a new world of safe and healthy schools.

2

Safe and Healthy Schools in Preschool Settings

CHRIS SWANSON, EDD

For the average individual, life course is determined by less than 5 percent of an entire life span. Physiological, emotional, and cognitive development from conception to age five significantly impact later health, social relationships, academic and work performance, and ultimately, societal contributions. While biology plays a role, it is well established that the experiences a child has during early childhood can have a critical influence on the trajectory of their life. With nearly 60 percent of US children under age five enrolled in some form of nonparental care (Committee for Economic Development [CED] 2019), these settings have a profound impact on a child's development. Whether it is through strong child engagement, targeted early intervention, or protection from the adverse effects associated with trauma and child maltreatment, high-quality early childhood education and care (ECEC) embodies practices and structures that contribute profoundly to a child's development and well-being (Cannon et al. 2018). This impact continues beyond the given moment and is seen in an individual's later earning potential, better interpersonal relationships, reduced likelihood of incarceration, and greater health and life expectancy (McCoy et al. 2017). While there are many variations in the specific components that constitute quality, there is consensus that three conditions broadly contribute to the greatest child outcomes: (1) interpersonal interactions between adults and children; (2) safe, engaging, and developmentally appropriate environments, inclusive of curriculum and materials, that are designed to stimulate the child; and (3) an effective operational model that ensures qualified and competent personnel are consistent in a child's life, that there are sufficient resources—from diapers to learning materials, that suitable adult-to-child ratios are maintained, and that families are treated as partners to ensure continuous nurturing of the child's growth across home and school (National Association for the Education of Young Children [NAEYC] 2019; Wechsler et al. 2016). In short, higher-quality ECEC advances a child's physical and emotional safety; enables positive cognitive, motoric, and social-emotional development; and promotes greater lifelong success than lesser-quality settings and experiences.

State of Early Childhood Education and Care

Despite significant research that demonstrates the positive effects on children who receive ECEC that implement the above elements, the US childcare landscape remains a patchwork of regulations, quality, and availability that often exacerbates inequities by socioeconomics and race. As high-quality ECEC are safe and healthy environments that instill lifetime benefits, the need to ensure all children are accessing these environments must be a national priority. The reality is even before the COVID-19 pandemic, America's ECEC system was in crisis: fragmented and inconsistent, held back by roots in classism and racism. The pandemic simultaneously demonstrated how critical ECEC is to family well-being and the entire economy while also revealing the system's fragility. Prepandemic studies found that large swatches of the United States were childcare deserts, with more than three eligible children per available slot (CED 2019). Models projected a loss of up to 4.5 million slots nationwide when ECEC programs were closed due to the pandemic (Soto 2020). One out of five ECEC workers lost their job during the pandemic, and the US ECEC workforce remains one of the last industries to recover to prepandemic levels (Crouse et al. 2023). Women were disproportionately forced out of the workforce to care for children who lacked access to ECEC or school during COVID-19. An exacerbation of the already too short supply of quality ECEC will either permanently reduce family income and earnings, forcing more families into poverty, or create a greater reliance on illegal, unregulated, or unsupervised custodial care situations that do little for imparting the benefits of quality ECEC and put children at risk.

What follows is an examination of the relationship between quality, safe, and beneficial ECEC. A description of what constitutes such environments, their importance, and what is needed to ensure safe ECEC for the millions of children served by them will culminate with a call to action to scale up what is currently being done well and what is still needed to ensure all children are served by safe and efficacious ECEC.

Quality ECEC Is Safe ECEC

The concept of safety in the context of ECEC speaks not to preventing every scrape and tumble but to larger constructs of child well-being: the prevention of abuse, neglect, and serious injury; promotion of positive social, emotional, physical, and cognitive development; and mitigating the effects of adverse childhood experiences (ACEs), as mentioned in chapter 4. The focus on these outcomes gets enshrined in several elements of a regulated childcare system. Licensure typically serves as the baseline, with programs receiving governmental approval to operate based on meeting specific criteria. Initiatives like accreditation and quality rating go beyond licensure to recognize specific implemented practices known to promote the above outcomes.

As such, a growing trend to ensure early childhood programs demonstrate these components through practices and policies has become an increasing national priority. Quality Rating Improvement Systems (QRIS), more recently with some states substituting "Recognition" for "Rating," were developed as a means of defining and implementing effective practices conducive to positive child development and well-being. At present, every US state either has a QRIS or is working to implement one, with more than forty other countries having similar models. While there is not a national definition of early care and education quality, nor a universal model for how to measure, QRIS typically features the following elements:

1. *Program standards*—used to assign ratings to programs, often along a scale of levels reflecting the degree of implemented quality ele-

ments, which serve as a basis for communication to the public and targeted improvement for the program.

2. *Supports for programs and practitioners*—reflective of training, coaching, mentoring, and technical assistance designed to assist programs in increasing their quality.
3. *Financial incentives*—typically funding intended to encourage participation or reward programs that increase and sustain quality levels. Some states connect subsidies to reduce the cost of childcare for income-eligible families to enrollment in a QRIS-rated program—seeking to drive access to higher quality for the most in need populations of children.
4. *Quality assurance and monitoring*—the process by which the quality ratings are measured and validated to ensure the system is accurate and reliable.
5. *Consumer education*—the basis by which the importance of quality, and the specific demonstrated elements of a given program, are made available to the public to inform family choice when selecting care and early education for their child (Mitchell 2005).

Collectively, these elements influence ECEC programs toward implementing practices conducive to child well-being. Tout et al. (2017) conducted a meta-analysis of QRIS validation studies to find nearly 85 percent had the following common elements reflected in their program standards: adherence to licensing requirements, though there was variation about the allowance of none to certain types of violations; implementation of developmentally appropriate practices, including using positive behavioral responses and having other social-emotional supports; family supports, including resource sharing for social and health services; standards of staff training and credentialing; and an emphasis on child nutrition, such as through participation in the federal Child and Adult Care Food Program to provide free meals. While the findings showed commonality of inclusion in the standards, there was significant variability in the specific required evidence that programs needed to demonstrate meeting the standards. Likewise, twenty-three out of forty-one states that report their QRIS data through the publicly available QRIS Data Compendium utilizes a point or hybrid rating system. These models allow programs to achieve a rating by choosing certain elements of quality to demonstrate, valued with associated points, in order to achieve a total requisite score for a given rating level. The hybrid model allows a combination of certain required elements and point allocations, while a block system, utilized by seventeen states currently, requires demonstration of all required elements for a given level (QRIS Data Compendium 2022). With point and hybrid systems, it is less certain the programs are implementing each of the elements associated with child well-being. Still, thirty-one states explicitly require health and safety training as an element of QRIS workforce credentials for childcare providers and teachers (Sergi et al. 2017). These training courses cover typical areas of emergency preparedness and response, though not necessarily cardiopulmonary resuscitation training. They touch on hygiene and mandatory reporting of suspected abuse and highlight other traditional aspects of base licensing, such as appropriate adult supervision and interactions, reducing potential for harm from the environment by proper storage of chemicals or other dangerous objects, and safety procedures for child release, emergency contacts, and other operational policies. QRIS presume these elements are in place in the absence of a documented licensing violation or utilize third-party observation tools like the Environmental Rating Scales to corroborate implementation of procedures conducive to a safe and healthy environment. While these elements put a focus on the importance of the environment and procedures, it is the measured implementation of developmentally appropriate practices that elevate QRIS programs and strengthen their impact on a child's immediate and long-term well-being.

The National Association for the Education of Young Children (NAEYC) defines developmentally appropriate practices (DAP) as "methods that promote each child's optimal development and learning through a strengths-based, play-based approach to joyful, engaged learning" (NAEYC 2022). The implementation of DAP is considered a key marker of high-quality ECEC, with effective DAP promoting health and safety in the form of physical, social, emotional, and cognitive development (C. Brown et al. 2018).

In high-quality childcare and early education, DAP practices are in place to address children's social and emotional development. Multiple studies have established a link between aggressive and antisocial behaviors in young children as a precursor for continued challenging behavior throughout K–12 and later-life incidents of mental health and legal issues (Brennan et al. 2012; Dodge et al. 2015; Jones et al. 2015). It has been established that social and emotional delays and challenges occur in 10–20 percent of children aged two through five (Brauner and Stephens 2006; Egger and Angold 2006). A typical result is preschool-aged children are three times more likely to be expelled than children in K–12 (Gilliam and Shahar 2006), and this trend is more likely to impact Black children than their peers. Black boys make up 19 percent of the preschool enrollment, yet 41 percent of all preschool suspensions are Black males (Strauss 2020). These early expulsion and suspension experiences have lifetime effects: a preschool child who is suspended or expelled more than once before kindergarten is ten times more likely to not complete high school, have higher rates of academic failure, and be incarcerated (Williams and Yogman 2023); Council on School Health et al. 2013; Petras et al. 2011). Likewise, these suspended children are more likely to have serious health and negative social interactions as adults, with a reduced life span (Gilliam and Shahar 2006; Lamont et al. 2013). Developmentally appropriate practices, often requisite within QRIS, use positive behavioral strategies such as the pyramid model to address dysregulated behavior (Dunlap and Fox 2015). They also address a zero expulsion or suspension approach for young children (US Department of Health and Human Services and US Department of Education, 2023). These evidence-based strategies are designed to promote positive behaviors and strong social-emotional development that directly equate to child safety and wellness now and into the child's future.

High-quality ECEC programs not only implement strong pedagogy but they also actively integrate health and wellness services for children and families and implement practices to mitigate adverse childhood experiences. ACEs have been defined as negative life experiences; when exposed to at least four of these events in childhood, an individual's risk for later negative life outcomes across health and social status is significantly increased (Felitti et al. 2019). It was originally defined by categories of risk identified by exposure to abuse that is physical, emotional, and/or sexual to self or mother; living with substance abuse; family mental illness and suicide history; or exposure to the criminal justice system through family. Further research has demonstrated ACEs are even further reaching, with factors such as housing insecurity and hunger, toxic stress, and passive exposure to community violence generating the same long-term negative impacts (Boullier and Blair 2018; E. Lee et al. 2017; Shonkoff et al. 2012).

It is estimated that as many as one in four preschool-aged children experience ACEs (Jimenez et al. 2016), and numerous studies have shown that children with higher levels of ACEs experience greater difficulty in educational settings due to lack of engagement, dysregulated behaviors, absenteeism, and learning and development challenges (Lipscomb et al. 2021; Zeng et al. 2019). Therefore, it is imperative that effective ECEC programs implement practices to mitigate ACEs as much as possible. The US Centers for Disease Control and Prevention (CDC) notes "Ensuring Strong Start for Children" as one of its three essential ACEs prevention and mitigation strategies (Houry and Mercy 2019). Specially, the agency notes success of home-visiting programs like the Nurse-Family Partnership (NFP) program, where trained nurses enter the home to mentor, guide, and observe parenting practices, which has shown a 48 percent reduction in rates of child abuse and neglect (Olds et al. 1997; Sama-Miller et al. 2017). Home-visiting and other parental support strategies are a hallmark of quality ECEC programs. Additionally, use of developmentally appropriate practices that teach strong social-emotional learning skills, cultivates positive cognitive and physical development, and provides stability and consistency for children has been shown to help offset negative impacts of ACEs on these domains (J. Love et al. 2005; Reynolds et al. 2007). A landmark fifteen-year longitudinal study followed individuals with high ACE scores (more than four risk factors) who experienced quality ECEC through the Chicago Child-Parent Center (CPC) program. These children showed significant gains over peers in school performance and completion, less grade retention or need for special education services, and fewer incidents of behavioral concerns and incarceration (Reynolds et al. 2001). All things considered, access to quality ECEC has been shown to reduce incidents of abuse and neglect (Fortson et al. 2016). In part, this is attributed to reducing parental stress by ensuring the children have a safe place to receive care that reduces the burden on families, enabling better economic conditions for the family by allowing income earners to be at work while the children receive care. There is a growing body of evidence that suggests explicit trauma-informed care practices employed by ECEC professionals can be a decisive factor in improved outcomes.

The Substance Abuse and Mental Health Services Administration (SAMHSA) defined trauma as "an event, series of events, or set of circumstances experienced by an individual as physically or emotionally harmful or life-threatening with lasting adverse effects on the individual's functioning and mental, physical, social, emotional, or spiritual well-being" (SAMHSA 2014, p. 7). Trauma-informed care (TIC) is defined as an approach to providing support services that are accessible, appropriate, responsive, and prevents re-traumatization (Institute on Trauma and Trauma-Informed Care 2015). TIC is characterized by five core principles: safety, choice, collaboration, trustworthiness, and empowerment. Children who are exposed to trauma, from direct victimization of abuse to secondary exposure in their environments, demonstrate impaired brain physiology than peers who did not have these negative experiences. Exposure to trauma creates multiple physical changes: constant stress responses produce chemicals that alter the brain's structure and functioning, leading to less developed behavioral regulation and other executive functioning that impacts learning (van der Kolk et al. 2005). At the same time, as children's brains also develop through experiences, the lack of positive adult-child interactions leaves children who have experienced toxic stress less trusting of adults or bereft of typical positive adult-child models that promote a child's self-confidence, sense of self, and ability to self-regulate (Stubenbort et al. 2010). In short, a child who has been failed by the adults in their life learns to be less trusting, less secure in their feelings, less confident, and less safe in their world. This puts them at high risk for repeated victimization and greater likelihood of growing into perpetrators of abuse themselves (Merrick et al. 2019). Recognizing this critical issue, a growing number of states have begun to integrate TIC practices into their ECEC initiatives. The National Center on Early Childhood Quality Assurance (NCECQA), a federally supported training and dissemination of best-practices entity, reported trauma-informed care as the fastest-growing category of request support by states in 2019 (NCECQA 2019). That was prepandemic, and COVID-19 only created an even greater universal trauma for all children, exasperating other underlying concerns for those children already at risk of ACEs. Beyond training for personnel, early childhood mental health, including referral and direct services for children, has also become a routine element of quality childcare. A growing area of focus is the emerging relationship between the childcare workforce's mental health and their ability to provide effective services to children. Jeon et al. (2021) examined a series of peer-reviewed studies published between 2005 and 2019 which revealed a direct correlation between childcare professionals' reported levels of well-being and child-level outcomes of children in their care. Childcare professionals with higher indices of stress, physical and emotional illness, and job dissatisfaction were more likely to suspend and expel children, were more likely to have children with lower measured engagement and school performance, and were more likely to turn-over, creating disruption in continuity of care for the children—another factor associated with child-experienced stress. What was clear is that of teachers who were serving a similar population of children, those associated with higher-quality schools—even when exposed to the same environmental challenges as their colleagues in lower-quality programs—reported greater levels of well-being. Factors associated with greater well-being included strong workplace relationships and support networks, fair wage and compensation, good working conditions, disciplinary efficacy—often associated with administrative support, and perceived professionalism of their role. As higher-quality ECEC is often associated with initiatives like QRIS and accreditation, greater staff training, access to higher government funding to help improve wages, and strong administrative practices, it was hypothesized that these are the conditions that make the difference in quality ECEC.

Collectively, quality ECEC utilizes standards of developmentally appropriate practice that meet the emotional, physical, and cognitive needs of children; they require trainings for effective health, safety, and implemented programming that help children thrive; and they serve as connectors for families to additional resources and supports shown to mitigate negative impacts of ACEs and trauma. What follows is an examination of several validated quality ECEC programs and the associated child and societal benefits.

The Importance of Quality

President Lyndon B. Johnson's War on Poverty would directly lead to the creation of Head Start, a comprehensive child development program that looked at parental and child interventions to meet the needs of impoverished children. Informed by scientific evidence with expertise from the likes of Dr. Robert Cooke, a pediatrician at Johns Hopkins Hospital, and Dr. Edward Zigler, a professor of psychology and director of the Child Study Center at Yale University, Head Start integrated multiple critical ECEC elements: (1) governmental investment for ensuring consistency and quality practices; (2) a holistic approach to all elements that influence child development—from child engagement through robust curricula implemented by trained professionals to ensuring safety, health, and nutritional needs of the child and family were paramount; (3) the acknowledgment that positive child development was a partnership—between school, family, and child as well as the community; and (4) programming responsive to the child's cultural and linguistic heritage (Office of Head Start 2023; Congress.gov 2007).

Early Childhood Landscape

Basic health and safety begin with licensure to operate a childcare program, yet this system is woefully inconsistent across the country. Licensure requirements are highly variable, with twenty-seven states allowing levels of unregulated childcare (Fischer and Orlowski 2020). This is particularly concerning since most deaths in childcare occur in these types of environments. The last major study to examine deaths in care found 1,362 deaths in childcare facilities between 1985 and 2003 (Wrigley and Dreby

2005), with 1,030 of those occurring in either unregulated or illegal childcare facilities. The American Academy of Pediatrics estimates based on population data that 9 percent of all sudden infant death syndrome (SIDS) would naturally occur within childcare programs, but that number is closer to 20 percent (Moon 2016). Recent state-specific analyses are more alarming. The *Washington Post* investigated a decade of Virginia childcare deaths and found of sixty children who died, 75 percent occurred in unregulated but legally operating childcare programs, with 25 percent of the deaths due to abuse (Fallis and Brittain 2014). Investigative reporting in Indiana, Missouri, and Texas confirmed similar trends of the majority of childcare deaths occurring in unregulated environments (Cambria 2011; Lundstrum 2018; Weddle 2014). To answer whether regulations make a difference, Minnesota saw a spike of child deaths in care in 2012, which resulted in improved health and safety standards for both licensing and their QRIS system. When implemented, deaths fell to an all-time low (Schrade 2013). There are multiple factors that contribute to these outcomes: (1) Per the federal Child Care Development Fund block grants that states rely on to largely fund their childcare systems, fingerprinting and background checks of personnel who both work with children, but also those who live in the house where licensed childcare is provided from the provider's home, are mandatory; (2) both scheduled and random inspections of facilities are routine within licensed programs; and (3) families have recourse to report concerns and access to data about incidents of neglect, abuse, and deaths, as well as other licensing violations, through federally required state consumer education websites. But these safeguards are only in place for licensed programs and enforceable for states that accept federal monies; even with these protections in place, licensing only represents the baseline provision. Licensing tends to focus on the physical environment and basic operational structures such as hygiene practices, leaving the adult-child interactions, specific curriculum implementations, and other contributions to physical, emotional, and cognitive development for others to monitor. This is what gave rise to QRIS and program accreditation standards; yet even here, leveraging QRIS to address ACEs and trauma, key predictors for long-term negative outcomes are an emerging need as previously described (Samuels 2022). The reality is that despite effective licensure and quality initiatives, a significant number of children are not benefiting from these structures.

In 2019, of the 7.9 million US children aged three and four, 52 percent and 67 percent, respectively, were in some form of external childcare or preschool setting for an average of 26.7 hours per week (Hussar et al. 2020). The US ECEC landscape remains a dizzying array of program types, hours, and quality, with the latter often delineated by economic standing. Pre-COVID-19, there were approximately 3.8 million ECEC settings serving 12.1 million children from birth to age five—roughly 58.7 percent of the 20 million US children under age five (CED 2019). The vast majority of childcare is provided in the home of a nonparental individual, comprising nearly 97 percent of all available care (Hussar et al. 2020). Family child care (FCC) can be licensed or legally operate unregulated programs that provide care for children of mixed ages, out of the home of a paid childcare provider. Most states have enrollment caps, but that number varies across the country and by the age of children. FCC accounts for 27.5 percent of all home-based care, employing about 1,037,000 people before the pandemic. About 11 percent of children under age five, more heavily weighted toward infants and toddlers, were enrolled in FCC (National Survey of Early Care and Education Project Team [NSECEPT] 2016). That leaves the bulk of home-based care (72.5%) to be a mixture of friends, families, neighbors, and in-home nannies who provide informal, often unregulated supervision for pay or no cost, of more than 5 million children. FCC and home-based care are heavily utilized because of cost, flexibility in hours to match work schedules, and parental comfort with the provider, but most of these arrangements are not licensed or regulated, let alone supported or monitored for any implemented standards of quality. As described earlier, deaths and serious injuries occur more frequently in unregulated environments.

Center-based childcare ("centers") typically refers to half- or full-day programs that tend to mirror more traditional work hours for parents. Centers are often privately owned, with several corporate models, though there are examples of public-private partnerships wherein independently managed centers are co-located at a school or other public institution. Most centers are licensed or regulated, though some states reduce the normal setup or monitoring processes for license-exempt programs, often located within religious institutions. Centers provide care for about 2.4 million children; the majority are aged three to five years, though many offer services for infants and toddlers (NSECEPT 2016). Adding to the fragmented nature of US ECEC are inconsistent definitions of program types. The distinction between centers, preschools, and pre-kindergarten is one such example. US preschools, inclusive of formalized programming for children from age three to kindergarten entry, which has varying age cutoffs by state, are often classrooms within centers. The most practical distinction for centers is by funding entity. In that regard here, centers include standalone private preschools and tuition-based programs offering care from infant to kindergarten. As such, this collective definition of centers constitutes approximately 3 percent of childcare, serving 3.5 million children and employing about 1 million professionals (NSECEPT 2016). Head Start, a governmentally funded ECEC for children in poverty, enrolled 873,019 children in FY2019 (Administration for Children and Families [ACF] 2019). The US poverty rate for children under age five is 15.5 percent, or nearly 1.87 million children (Haider 2021), so Head Start and its infant and toddler analog served about 47 percent of eligible children.

Public preschools are typically school-year programs operated by local school systems, mostly serving children aged four, though there has been a growing movement to expand to age three. Traditionally funded at the state and local levels, admission criteria are left to the school system. To increase availability, federal funding has focused on "Universal Pre-K," with a goal of getting every three- and four-year-old into a high-quality Pre-K program. In many states, this funding is disbursed across public-school-operated Pre-K classrooms and community-based private childcare if all meet defined criteria. Even with these efforts, in the 2018–19 school year, only 37 percent of four-year-olds and 6 percent of three-year-olds were enrolled in publicly funded preschool programs (Friedman-Krauss et al. 2020), at a cost of $7.6 billion (ACF 2020).

In total, 48 percent of American three-year-olds and 33 percent of four-year-olds were not in any form of reported care or education in 2018–19;

yet during this same time period, the number of total eligible children compared to the supply of available slots was 3:1, with only 16 percent of households reporting they were able to provide full-time parental care (CED 2019). This means many families rely on informal, illegal, or other forms of unregulated care that can have questionable quality and could potentially be deadly.

In short, the environments in which a child spends their formative time prior to kindergarten play a significant role in their development. As such, it is imperative that these environments, and the professionals who work in them, maximize best practices to help children and their families realize the full benefits of this critical period. Unfortunately, barriers such as a fragmented set of licensing regulations, low pay and education levels of the workforce, politics, and systemic challenges of societal poverty and racism conspire against a consistent national model of effective and safe early childhood education. At the same time, K–12 school accountability reforms have created downward pressure on preschool settings to increase academic preparedness—often at the cost of developmentally appropriate practices that would normally engender social-emotional and other well-being outcomes, which becomes a contributor for later mental health and behavioral challenges. The benefits of quality ECEC are known, long-lasting, and when measured appropriately, indicative of long-term success across multiple positive life outcomes. The real barrier to fully implement a comprehensive and effective US ECEC system remains perceived costs that are rooted in issues of classism, racism, and the role of government in education.

Investing in Impact

The average annual cost per child for Head Start services is $10,000 (ACF 2020). Ironically, this is the least expensive exemplar ECEC model, with calculated costs for private-pay, high-quality ECEC ranging from $15,840 to $27,120 per child based on age and setting (Workman and Jessen-Howard 2018). For the most part, this is not nearly what is being paid for in ECEC, and that is already cost prohibitive. The US Administration for Children and Families defines childcare affordability as 7 percent of household income, but that rate is only achieved by the wealthiest families. On average, childcare costs account for 30 percent of a family's income, with not nearly enough governmental subsidy available to address the needs, as government subsidizing of tuition costs only benefits about 15 percent of all eligible children (Jessen-Howard et al. 2020; Ullrich et al. 2019).

The benefit of subsidized care also varies wildly, as the actual amount allocated to a family is a function of a market rate and does not consider the affordability formulas as a function of household income. Since most states do not mandate private childcare providers to accept subsidy vouchers, and those that do tend to fall on the lower end of quality measurement metrics, achieving the known benefits for economically disadvantaged children to have access to high-quality ECEC continues to elude this country (Ullrich et al. 2019). In fact, out of all industrialized nations, the United States ranks last in terms of affordability and access by percentage of child population.

There is no room for programs or families to absorb more cost. The average childcare worker makes $23,471 a year (McLean et al. 2021). The 2019 US federal poverty level was $25,750 for a family of four. One in seven childcare workers, predominantly women, are already living below the federal poverty level, and less than 25 percent of the workforce has paid health insurance or any type of leave benefits (Gould and Blair 2020). These statistics play out in a field that employs 2.5 Black and Hispanic women for every White woman, adding to the inequity of impact (McLean et al. 2021).

High-quality ECEC needs to be a public spending priority. Multiple economic models calculate a return on investment of 13.7 percent per annum for every dollar spent on quality ECEC (García et al. 2016). Costs for health care, incarceration, and K–12 interventions like special education have been shown to be reduced, while income and tax revenues increase because of quality ECEC. Models show a direct subsidy of about $42 billion per year would allow all children up to two hundred times the federal poverty level—approximately 50 percent of all US children—to receive completely free ECEC with the current system (Whitehurst 2019). A far greater investment is needed to ensure all programs are high quality, including paying wages in line with K–12 education, while maintaining flexibility of locations and hours necessary to meet parents where they live and work. Gould and Blair (2020) estimate the costs of this model to be closer to $495 billion to provide every American child free, high-quality ECEC. While ten times larger than current public spending, ECEC investments trigger multiple cost offsets. Beyond the 13.7 percent return on investment previously mentioned from all the developmental benefits, such an approach generates about $115 billion in currently lost wages and subsequent tax revenues from parents able to work and comparable K–12 wages for childcare workers. Investments in quality ECEC are not just good for children and families, they make good sense economically. The question should not be about whether the investment is worth it, but how can all children participate in high-quality ECEC programs?

The Future

Quality ECEC is a core tenet of American life. It promotes strong child development that yields a lifetime of improved outcomes, not just for the child but all of society. Safe and healthy schools begin with quality ECEC experiences. As such, the United States needs to invest in the infrastructure to support this: (1) a standardized national data system with common definitions of program types and modernized data collection and reporting mechanisms, including all incidents of neglect, abuse, serious injury, and death; (2) consistent and enforced licensing standards for all ECEC; and (3) public information campaigns on the benefits of using regulated, quality ECEC.

The ECEC workforce needs wages and benefits that ensure no worker is in poverty and is equipped with the professional knowledge to be successful. This requires a comprehensive and realistic approach to building the professional skills and behaviors of the workforce by increasing their confidence and competence via a mixed model of formal and informal professional learning paths.

National common QRIS standards need to emphasize children's holistic physical, emotional, cognitive, and social development, with particular emphasis on ensuring trauma-informed care and developmentally appropriate practice with local flexibility in curriculum and materials. Examination of school readiness needs to broaden to the entire developmental trajectory of a child—not simply their ability to perform on state reading and math tests. Leveraging common data systems, longitudinal analyses methodologies need to measure long-term benefits in health, education, behavior, economic, and social well-being outcomes.

Barriers to access need to be removed by reducing cost and increasing quality ECEC availability via government investment. Quality ECEC needs to be free for any family earning up to 200 percent of the federal poverty level. Subsidies and tax deductions for tuition costs of licensed, quality-rated ECEC should then cap all other families' direct out-of-pocket costs to 7 percent of household income. This will create incentives to flow enrollments into programs that help to stabilize the ECEC market while ensuring all children, regardless of economic status, benefit.

The United States prides itself on a myth of Horatio Alger self-advancement through achieving success via academic hard work; however, educational systems have historically perpetuated class status too often correlated by race. High-quality ECEC is proven to lead to healthier, productive, safer, and better lives for citizens. Ensuring a quality ECEC system is nothing short of making good on the words enshrined in America's founding of equality and "life, liberty, and the pursuit of happiness."

Conclusion

Prioritizing access to high-quality ECEC should not be a political issue. Investments pay for themselves. Benefits are seen in improved health, safety, long-term wealth, and societal contributions, with more significant gains for children in poverty. Since that is too often synonymous with Black, Hispanic, and Indigenous children in America, investments in quality ECEC address generational systemic racial inequity. High-quality ECEC is one part of the antidote, and it is one that has been known for centuries.

3

School-Based Suicide Prevention Interventions for Cultivating Mental Health Safety

HOLLY C. WILCOX, PHD

About 20 to 25 percent of school-aged youths have a mental health concern that impairs their social, academic, or family functioning, and 80 percent of chronic mental disorders begin in childhood (Merikangas et al. 2010). The most common mental health conditions in school-aged youths are anxiety disorders, depression, behavioral disorders, and attention-deficit/hyperactivity disorder (ADHD). National surveys have shown the rates of depression and anxiety have been increasing in the United States, especially among girls, and with the largest increases after 2011 (Substance Abuse and Mental Health Services Administration [SAMHSA] 2018; Keyes et al. 2020). Despite the increase in rates of depression, there have not been increases in mental health treatment (Mojtabai et al. 2016).

Following accidents or unintentional injuries, suicide is the second leading cause of death for children ages ten to fourteen (Centers for Disease Control and Prevention [CDC] 2023), and recent epidemiological trends indicate that suicidal ideation and attempts among children and adolescents are on the rise (CDC 2023). Youth suicide rates have risen over 60 percent in the last decade, and suicide remains the second leading cause of death for youths aged 12–19 years, responsible for approximately 1 in 5 deaths in that age group (CDC, 2023).

Factors Associated with Suicide

In the United States, the age of suicidal ideation onset increases slowly until the age of twelve years, and then dramatically increases between the ages of twelve and seventeen (CDC 2021). The prevalence of suicide is about five times higher in adolescents ages fifteen to nineteen years of age (10.5 per 100,000 persons) compared to children ages ten to fourteen (2.6 per 100,000) (CDC 2023), which has been attributed to the emergence of psychiatric symptoms and disorders during adolescence (Nock et al. 2013). Psychiatric risk factors such as depression, anxiety, and alcohol and drug use increase the risk of suicide in youths of all ages (Nock et al. 2013; Brent et al. 1999). These disorders and their symptoms are not uncommon in youths younger than fourteen years of age (Sheftall et al. 2016). Stressful events such as family or school crises or disciplinary events (Sheftall et al. 2016; Fergusson et al. 2000), interpersonal or community violence exposure (Sheftall et al. 2016; Fergusson et al. 2000; Soole et al. 2015; Dervic et al. 2008), and hopelessness, low self-esteem, aggression, and impulsivity are also linked with risk of suicide in youths (O'Leary et al. 2006; Thompson et al. 2005; Pfeffer et al. 1998; Hawton et al. 2012; Tomek et al. 2015). Connectedness with family, friends, school, and the community are strong protective factors for suicidal behaviors (defined as suicidal ideation, attempts, and suicide) in youths (Borowsky, Resnick, et al. 1999; Czyz et al. 2012; Borowsky, Ireland, et al. 2001; O'Donnell et al. 2003). Most adolescents who experience suicidal ideation move from ideation to having a suicide plan (63%) within the first year of onset, and then among those, a larger majority (88%) move from ideation to attempt (Nock et al. 2013), again underscoring the importance of early intervention. In addition to the immediate effects on the individual, suicidal behaviors are devastating for family, friends, schools, and communities and warrant urgent public health action.

The epidemiology of youth suicide has been changing over time in the United States. Suicidal behaviors vary across race, sex, income, and sexual identity. Although Indigenous youth have the highest rates of suicide, the suicide death rate among Black youth is increasing faster than any other racial/ethnic group (Congressional Black Caucus 2019). The 2021 National Youth Risk Behavior Survey of high school students found that 14 percent of Black high school students reported making a suicide attempt in the prior year compared to 11 percent of Hispanic students and 9 percent of White students (CDC 2021a). The rate of suicide in children ages five to twelve years is about two times higher for Black children compared to White children among both males and females (Bridge et al. 2018). Among Black youth who were followed from first grade into adulthood in Baltimore, Maryland, the peak in incidence of suicidal ideation occurred in seventh grade (ages 12 to 13 typically) with rates of 9 percent (Musci et al. 2016). Unlike the increases in rates among older teens seen in the overall population, a steady decline in ideation was seen in subsequent grades for Baltimore youth (Musci et al. 2016). This data underscores the importance of intervening at the youngest age feasible.

Research also consistently shows that female youth have higher rates of suicidal ideation and attempts compared to males; however, males have higher rates of suicide (Miranda-Mendizabal et al. 2019). Sexual identity is also a very strong risk factor for victimization and suicidal behaviors in youth such that lesbian, gay, bisexual, transgender, and questioning youth show significantly elevated risk of suicidal behaviors compared to heterosexual youth (Johns et al. 2020; Garofalo et al. 1999). Sexual minority youth often identify as such in the early stages of puberty, which could be associated with increases in suicidal behaviors during this developmental period. Sociodemographic factors such as socioeconomic disadvantage and county poverty concentration have also been shown to increase the risk of suicidal behaviors in adolescents (Yildiz et al. 2019; Hoffmann et al. 2020). According to the CDC, emergency department visits for suspected suicide attempts among persons aged twelve to seventeen increased 31 percent during the COVID-19 pandemic compared with before the pandemic. This was especially pronounced for adolescent girls, whose suspected suicide attempt emergency department visits were 50.6 percent higher than before the pandemic (Yard et al. 2021).

Prevention Programs and Legislation, and the Role of Schools

Schools can and must play a vital role in mental health because the first onset of mental illness typically occurs in childhood or adolescence, and children and teens spend a significant amount of time in school. School officials can help identify students at risk, deliver risk assessment or evaluation, enact preventive and treatment interventions, refer to community-based providers, and provide support in the aftermath of suicide. Education policies are increasingly calling for expansion of school-based health efforts (American Foundation for Suicide Prevention [AFSP] et al. 2019). Evidence-based school intervention programming, crisis response, and postvention policies are key to addressing the persistent increasing trends in youth suicide. To support the development and improvement of school-based interventions, the AFSP has developed the *Model School District Policy on Suicide Prevention*, which provides a framework that can be customized to meet the unique needs of each school district (2019).

Many states have recently established laws mandating or encouraging the training of school personnel, including teachers, in suicide prevention as well as the development of districtwide policies and programs (AFSP 2020). Currently, there is a great deal of variation in both the quality, content, intensity, and costs of the training and programs, and limited data exist on how well policies are implemented. Thirteen states have legislation in place for annual suicide prevention training for teachers, administrators, counselors, and other specialists who provide services to students. An additional nineteen states (and Washington, DC) also have state-mandated training but not annually. Suicide prevention training is encouraged but not required in fifteen states.

Most students participate in health education in school, which is intended to address social and emotional health, safety, and injury prevention. Unfortunately, schools are often not provided guidance on which programs to select, based on the characteristics of their student population, program evidence of effectiveness, and program sustainability potential. Program fidelity and quality of implementation is not emphasized or encouraged. In addition, many schools have programming that is a one-time effort and not sustained.

Although most existing school suicide prevention programming is directed at high school students, the national suicide morbidity and mortality data show that only focusing on high school is too late for some students to fully benefit. However, schools and parents sometimes feel unprepared for how to address suicidal thoughts and behavior, especially in elementary and middle school students. In addition, many of the existing school-based programs aim to identify students after the crisis has already started (which is also too late).

The US Surgeon General (Office of the Surgeon General 2021) has a call to action to implement the National Suicide Prevention Strategy, including building skills (e.g., coping, problem solving) and resilience by increasing social connectedness, identifying students at risk for suicide, and supporting help seeking and access to effective mental health care (US Department of Health and Human Services and the Office of the Surgeon General 2021). Universal school-based interventions are those that are offered to the entire population, and thus do not stigmatize at-risk students by identifying them for a targeted intervention (Calear and Christensen 2010). Universal programs also have the potential to benefit large numbers of students who may not be symptomatic at the time of the intervention but may otherwise go on to have problems without the intervention (Robinson et al. 2013).

J. J. Mann and colleagues (2021), in a systematic review of suicide prevention programs, found that school-based programs directed at teaching all students how to help a friend with mental health concerns and crises were found to prevent student suicide attempts, whereas programs only training adults in schools to identify students at risk did not find benefit on suicidal behaviors. These types of peer-to-peer programs can be embedded into the standard health education curriculum, with the goal of building mental health literacy and skills while demystifying/destigmatizing mental health care.

Enhancing the knowledge, attitudes, and behaviors of adolescent peer groups is an important approach for suicide prevention in youths. The teen Mental Health First Aid (tMHFA) (Hart, Morgan, et al. 2018) curriculum is a classroom-based training program to teach adolescents how to assist their friends experiencing mental health concerns including suicidal behaviors. The program was tested in Australian high schools and, in a randomized controlled trial, was found to increase adolescents' recognition of peers at risk for suicide and improve confidence in supporting a suicidal peer (Hart, Cropper, et al. 2020). This program was adapted for use in the United States and is being tested, with very promising early results.

The Youth Aware of Mental health (YAM) program is included in the CDC's *Preventing Suicide: A Technical Package of Policies, Programs, and Practices* (Stone et al. 2017) and was one of three programs evaluated in the Saving and Empowering Young Lives in Europe (SEYLE) randomized controlled trial (RCT) in the European Union among 11,110 students (ages 14–16) from 168 schools randomly selected in eleven European Union countries (Wasserman, Hoven et al. 2015; Wasserman, Carli, et al. 2010; Carli et al. 2013). The evaluation of YAM used structured assessments composed of established scales administered to students at baseline, and at a three-month and twelve-month follow-up. YAM, a classroom-based skill-building intervention, was associated with a 50 percent reduction in suicide attempts and a 30 percent reduction in incident cases of moderate or severe depression at twelve months follow-up (Wasserman, Hoven, et al. 2015). Further, the YAM program was well received by students, parents, and school personnel as demonstrated through high rates of participation and satisfaction (Wasserman, Hoven, et al. 2015). In an uncontrolled within-subjects design assessing the feasibility and outcomes of delivering YAM to ninth and tenth graders in Texas and Montana, Lindow, Hughes, South, Gutierrez, and colleagues (2020) found that the YAM intervention was feasible to adapt for United States high schools, implement, and evaluate with a high degree of program satisfaction. Depression and anxiety scores decreased after YAM implementation in this pilot study in Montana (Lindow, Hughes, South, Gutierrez, et al. 2020). In a study of 436 adolescents in Montana and Texas, significant increases were found before to three months after YAM in three of five help-seeking behaviors, along with improved mental health literacy and decreased mental health–related stigma. However, intent to seek help was unchanged (Lindow, Hughes, South, Minhajuddin, et al. 2020). Although both YAM and tMHFA are designed for high school students, efforts are currently underway to adapt these programs for middle school students.

The Need for Earlier Interventions

The Good Behavior Game (GBG) is a universal preventive intervention carried out in first- and second-grade classrooms (Barrish et al. 1969). GBG is precisely aimed at aggressive, disruptive behavior. The core elements of GBG are to (1) define rules: teachers with children define rules for classroom behavior; (2) establish teams: students in classrooms are divided into three or four teams evenly matched in terms of behavior; (3) play the game: during the game, the teacher counts rule infractions (the game is played no more than five minutes to start); (4) announce winners: all teams can win the game; and (5) distribute rewards: social praise and rewards (e.g., blow bubbles or dance party for thirty seconds).

The first-generation GBG randomized prevention trial was conducted in Baltimore City Public Schools in 1985–87 among two consecutive cohorts. Cohort one started first grade in 1985, and cohort two started first grade in 1986. Cohort one had increased mentoring and monitoring of teachers implementing the GBG. In this trial, the GBG and Mastery Learning, two separate interventions, were compared to standard-setting classrooms internal and external to the intervention schools. Cohort one males in the high aggression trajectory showed significantly lower slopes of aggressive and disruptive behavior sustained through seventh grade (and sustained for females in the highest aggression trajectory through grade four) (Kellam, Rebok, et al. 1994; Kellam, Ling, et al. 1998; Petras et al. 2008). By young adulthood (i.e., age 19–21), there was a reduction in the rates of antisocial personality disorder, drug and alcohol abuse/dependence diagnoses and tobacco use (Kellam, Brown, et al. 2008), the use of school-based mental health services, antisocial personality disorder (Petras et al. 2008), and suicidal ideation and attempts (Wilcox et al. 2008). GBG impact was greatest in students with the highest levels of aggression and cohort one, indicating that GBG requires ongoing training and monitoring of teachers to achieve full impact (Kellam, Brown, et al. 2008). Bradshaw and colleagues (2009) found that the GBG was associated with higher scores on standardized achievement tests, greater odds of high school graduation and college attendance, and reduced odds of special education service use. Positive childhood peer relations partially explained the GBG-associated reduction of risk for suicide attempts (Newcomer et al. 2016).

In a very similar randomized trial in Europe, van Lier et al. (2005) also reported large reductions in antisocial behavior among children assigned to GBG with high baseline antisocial behavior. These reductions were partially mediated by improvements in peer relations. Children randomly assigned to GBG with high baseline antisocial behavior had more positive interactions with normatively developing boys and were less likely to be rejected by their peers, compared with control-group boys with high antisocial behavior. Witvliet et al. (2009) found that children assigned to GBG in kindergarten had significantly higher peer acceptance scores at the end of second grade compared with control-group children. Therefore, increases in peer acceptance partially mediated the reductions in externalizing behavior problems among GBG children. Menting et al. (2016) extended these findings to show that the GBG impact on second-grade internalizing problems (i.e., depressive and anxious symptoms) was also mediated by improved peer acceptance. Leflot et al. (2013) showed that the GBG resulted in a reduction in peer rejection among children with low levels of on-task behavior at baseline and that this decrease in peer rejection mediated the GBG impact on aggressive behavior.

Conclusion

Although some schools do not feel equipped to address student mental health challenges, there is ample evidence that mental health problems negatively impact learning and achievement, and school staff and peers are often the first individuals to recognize mental health problems in students. There are many actions schools could take to address these issues, including (1) enabling Medicaid reimbursement for schools to deliver mental health services like telemental health services, (2) training school mental health staff in how to conduct a suicide risk assessment and how to manage mental health crises, (3) embedding evidence-based school-based programming and mental health curricula that align with the National Health Education Standards, and (4) enhancing coordination and communication between schools and health care settings to address basic needs and mental health care by employing family navigators.

Coordinated, evidence-based, developmentally timed and stacked universal programs, such as GBG in elementary school, tMHFA and YAM in middle school and in high school are needed. Ideally, these stacked programs should also be conducted in the context of onsite school mental health services and proactive policies and workflow for how best to serve suicidal students as well as actions in the aftermath of student suicide to best address the increasing trends of suicidal thoughts and behaviors in students (STBs) in young adolescents. GBG, YAM, and tMHFA are evidence-based approaches that teach students different yet complementary developmentally appropriate skills. There is also a need to focus on sustainability and fidelity/quality of implementation of these approaches, as often these programs are not sustained in schools with high fidelity.

4

Asset-Based Approaches for Diverse Populations in Schools

BETH MARSHALL, DRPH, MPH, TERRINIEKA W. POWELL, PHD, AND ASARI OFFIONG, PHD, MPH

The terms *marginalized youth* and *vulnerable youth* refer to youths who are experiencing poverty, homelessness, involvement with the foster care or juvenile justice system, disconnection from work and school, pregnancy or parenting, challenges with their immigration status, or those young people who identify as racial, ethnic, or sexual minorities (Institute of Medicine and National Research Council 2015). These young people are more likely to experience negative, adverse experiences as they transition from childhood, to adolescence, and into adulthood (Sapiro and Ward 2019), which increases their vulnerability and likelihood of long-lasting negative outcomes. The vulnerability experienced by these young people is less solely a product of individual behaviors or circumstances and more a function of inequitable and unjust systems that prioritize punitive approaches and limit individuals' access to quality resources, services, and support. To advance health and academic equity, it is necessary to shift the narrative and explore opportunities that emphasize a young person's strengths and the assets within schools that can better support their well-being.

Schools and Vulnerable Youth

Schools have long been regarded as settings where youths can develop both academically and socially; however, as noted in chapter 6, that has not always been the case for vulnerable youth as their very expressions of being are often policed and punished by school administrators. Outside of the family unit, schools are a primary space where youths can access opportunities to develop cooperative social relationships and the skills needed to maintain these relationships, as well as develop connections to caring adults beyond the family unit (Twum-Antwi et al. 2020). Over the past two decades, the demographics in US public schools have become more racially diverse, with the percentage of Hispanic students increasing from 22 to 27 percent and those identifying with two or more races, increasing from 1 to 4 percent (Centers for Disease Control and Prevention [CDC] 2020b). In addition to those changes, US public schools have also seen a greater diversity in gender and sexual identity, with nearly 15 percent of students identifying as lesbian, gay, bisexual, queer, or transgender (LGBQT+) (CDC 2021a). Based on these shifts, schools need to be more expansive in meeting the needs of their diverse student population.

Given the vulnerability of marginalized youths, they have specific needs that impact their mental, physical, and academic well-being. These young people are more likely to have experienced trauma, which impedes their ability to focus during class, adjust to new environments, or feel a sense of belonging in their school. Some schools have met the challenge of expanding their services to address varying needs by offering physical and mental health care services onsite, supports for student social and emotional development, whole school interventions to ensure the school climate is safe and supportive for students who may have experienced or are currently experiencing family and/or community trauma, and resources to address other social determinants of health, such as food pantries onsite to address food insecurity. This is particularly noticeable in the Whole School, Whole Child, Whole Community model, which takes a holistic and coordinated approach to addressing the health and educational needs of students through multi-components, including physical education and physical activity, nutrition environment and services, health education, social and emotional climate, physical environment, health services, counseling, psychological and social services, employee wellness, community involvement, and family engagement (Lewallen et al. 2015).

There are still immense challenges faced by schools, including those related to social injustices, school safety, systemic racism, and discriminatory policies, to name a few. Schools can no longer be seen solely as an educational space, but rather one that sits at the intersection of individual-level experiences and societal mishaps—requiring more innovative approaches to addressing these challenges. Just as the needs of students and families have expanded, so too have the assets they bring into the school building. Assets, defined as strengths and protective factors that enhance a person's or community's ability to experience positive well-being and prevent health disparities (Morgan and Ziglio 2007), support positive outcomes among students. For example, community schools provide comprehensive support and resources that are selected to meet their students' and families' needs and interests, which are rooted in the partnering, understanding, and perspectives of the surrounding community. This chapter focuses on four asset-based approaches that are being used in schools to continually promote well-being for diverse students and families.

Asset-Based Approaches

Traditionally, approaches to working with students have often been based on a deficit model. We ask: What is the problem? What is lacking? Why are students failing? While focusing on the problem can lead to root causes or clear solutions, it disempowers and stigmatizes students. On the other hand, an *asset-based approach* is strengths-based and person-centered. It is rooted in the perspective that individuals have existing competencies, have available resources, and can and *should* be involved in the affairs of their well-being (Alliance for Children and Youth of Waterloo Region n.d.). Assets are factors that contribute to health promotion and can be leveraged to sustain long-lasting, positive outcomes. Asset-based approaches can be multilevel, in that there are factors across the individual, interpersonal, environmental, and systemic levels that support positive well-being. Considering that assets can be explored across levels, asset-based approaches nicely complement and fit within a prevention framework.

Asset-based approaches lead with the positive, which is particularly relevant when working with marginalized populations. In contrast to the carceral approach described in chapter 6, an asset-based approach invites teachers and other school personnel to consider strengths among groups usually thought of in terms of problems or failures (Luthar and Zelazo 2003). Youths, especially those from highly stressed communities or who are racially, sexually, and/or gender diverse, are often presented as problematic or labeled by their deficiencies (Doll and Lyon 1998). However, the language shift to asset based empowers and leads to trust, respect, and optimism among and between youths and adults. The positivity is evident in the language used to describe the eight core elements of asset-based approaches (figure 4.1):

1. *Emphasize capacity and intentionality*—starting from the premise that individuals have competencies and the ability to address issues related to their well-being
2. *Focus on personal relationships*—building rapport and establishing authentic relationships with youths
3. *Acknowledge contribution*—promoting successes and achievements
4. *Attend to the context/systems in which youths operate*—creating the awareness of and attention to social environments that frame and drive youth perspectives, decisions, and behaviors
5. *Invite meaningful contribution*—intentionally seeking and incorporating youths at various stages
6. *Provide opportunities for skill building*—exposing youths to new ideas and acquiring new strengths
7. *Recognize interrelationships*—acknowledging the intersectionality and dynamics between individuals
8. *Concentrate on solutions/potential*—limiting focus on root causes, but rather leveraging the strengths as opportunities for solutions (Alliance for Children and Youth of Waterloo Region n.d.).

While all asset-based approaches will not include all eight components mentioned above, each build on the value base that all youths have assets that can be leveraged for positive development and health. The four asset-based approaches this chapter highlights are (1) positive youth development, (2) trauma-informed approaches, (3) resilience building, and (4) critical

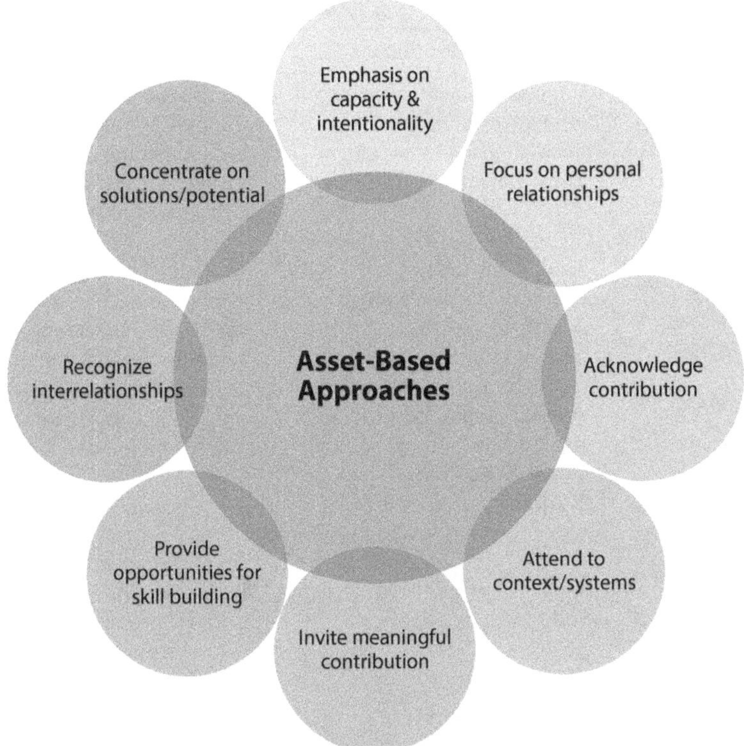

Figure 4.1 Eight core components of asset-based approaches.
Source: Adapted from *Strength-Based Approaches: Improving the Lives of Our Children and Youth*, © Alliance for Children and Youth of Waterloo Region

youth engagement. Each of these asset-based approaches can be utilized to effectively support the physical and mental health of vulnerable youth (table 4.1).

Positive Youth Development

Positive youth development is the process of moving beyond prevention of problem behaviors and into the realm of developing positive citizens. Practitioners develop and organize programs, support, and opportunities so that young people can reach their full potential. This approach was developed in the 1990s as a response to the long-standing beliefs that youths

Table 4.1 A Summary of Asset-Based Approaches

Approach	Definition	Examples in Schools
Positive Youth Development	Process of moving beyond prevention of problem behaviors and into realm of developing positive citizens	Harlem Lacrosse—integrated school-based sports youth development program that promotes learning and life skill development
Trauma-Informed Approaches	Recognizes the impact of trauma by developing program, organizational, or system support; recognizes the signs and symptoms of trauma; responds by integrating knowledge about trauma into policies, procedures, and practices; and seeks to actively resist re-traumatization	Restorative practices—a set of strategies used to build social capital and achieve social discipline through participatory learning and decision-making, enabling people to restore and build community
Resilience Building	Ability of people to successfully adapt and develop positive well-being in the face of adversity	Ayan Aba—intervention designed to the rate of growth of violence among Black youth
Critical Youth Engagement	Meaningful and sustained involvement of youth in activities that focus outside of themselves and bring their voices into community dialogue	Gender and sexuality alliances—student-run groups that bring together LGBTQ+ youth with allies to build a community and organize around LGBTQ+ issues

have problems that need to be fixed, and funding and programming are needed to fix these problems (i.e., dropout prevention, substance use prevention, and teen pregnancy prevention). As prevention science and prevention programs grew and researchers identified common predictors of the problem behaviors, the realization that thriving is not defined by the absence of problems set in and a paradigm shift toward a positive youth development approach fell under the tagline of "Problem-Free Is Not Fully Prepared" (Pittman et al. 2003). Lerner and colleagues (2005, 2013) set out to operationalize the attributes of thriving and developed the five Cs of competence, confidence, character, connection, and caring, leading to youth contributions, the sixth C of positive youth development.

The Six Cs are not the only model of positive youth outcomes. Several others touch on the same concepts but use different language, including Targeting Life Skills model, Essential Elements of 4-H Youth Development, Ready by 21, and the 40 Developmental Assets (Norman and Jordani 2006; Kress 2004; Yohalem et al. 2010; Benson and Scales 2009). While the language around outcomes may not be standard, the consensus regarding the variables that promote youth development was established in the early 2000s with the National Research Council and Institute of Medicine report outlining eight features with a focus on structure, safety, supports, and opportunities (National Research Council 2002). Evaluations of positive youth development programs identified the three most common features of effective youth-serving programs to be *positive and sustained relationships between youths and adults, activities that build important life skills*, and *opportunities for youths to use these life skills as both participants in and as leaders of valued community activities* (Blum 2003; Lerner 2004; Roth and Brooks-Gunn 2003). These three elements align with the core elements of asset-based approaches, including focusing on personal relationships, providing opportunities for skill building, and inviting meaningful participation.

Critics of positive youth development have suggested that the approach was developed for White middle-class youths and relies too heavily on support and opportunities without acknowledging the societal forces shaping a young person's world. This is particularly problematic for Black and Hispanic youths in neighborhoods with a history of disinvestment, as there is little recognition of the role of racism in limiting access to supports and opportunities. In response, Ginwright and Cammarota (2002) proposed a positive youth development model that incorporates a social justice approach to identifying and dismantling oppressive forces. Through critical analysis of these forces and social action, young people begin to heal from the racial and economic traumas they are challenged with each day. This adapted model of positive youth development aligns with the asset-based approach component of concentrating on solutions.

Schools aim to create an environment where every student can succeed regardless of race, gender, or other demographic characteristics. However, achievement gaps and disparities in school discipline have shown schools are not uniformly living up to this ideal for many students and that schools cannot ignore the community context their students bring with them into school buildings. Schools are an ideal place to employ the positive youth development approach because young people spend so many of their hours at school. The school environment includes academic and extracurricular activities, and therefore it has potential to impact the development of all six Cs (competence, confidence, character, connection, caring, contribution). Additionally, schools have the infrastructure to support a systems-level approach to youth development (Gomez and Ang 2007). Positive connections with peers and adults serve schools as well as adolescent development through enhancing students' sense of belonging in the building and their opportunities to develop interpersonal and intrapersonal skills (Pepler and Bierman 2018).

Example of Positive Youth Development in Schools: Harlem Lacrosse

Sports-based youth development programs operate in community or school contexts. They use specific sports to promote learning and life skill development (Perkins and Noam 2007). Harlem Lacrosse is an integrated school-based sports youth development program operating in five cities across the United States. Harlem Lacrosse's model includes school-based, full-day, year-round support for their students by placing a full-time staff member at school sites for each of its programs (i.e., one staff member for the girls' lacrosse program and one for the boys' lacrosse program). Harlem Lacrosse program directors maintain a constant presence in the lives of the student-athletes they serve. They act as tutors, mentors, and coaches to provide individualized attention that meets students where they are and helps them reach their full potential. In-school support is akin to a guidance counselor with a very targeted caseload. After-school support includes academic support in addition to lacrosse instruction, career exploration, social and emotional learning, service learning, and a focus on college pathways through college visits and admission supports. Harlem Lacrosse is shifting the racial dynamics in the sport of lacrosse by expanding opportunities and supports for students of color in urban settings who have historically been underrepresented in the sport. In addition, they prioritize hiring staff members who played NCAA Division I lacrosse and identify as persons of color. Nationally, 94 percent of their participants graduate high school compared to 85 percent of all students nationwide, 80 percent of economically disadvantaged students, 79 percent of Black students, and 81 percent of Latino/a and Hispanic students. In addition, 86 percent of participants enroll in college, and of those who enroll, 88 percent persist in college (Harlem Lacrosse 2020).

Trauma-Informed Approaches

A trauma-informed approach uses a universal precautions approach to support development and well-being (Substance Abuse and Mental Health Services Administration [SAMHSA] 2014). There are four core principles of a trauma-informed framework (also called the four Rs): (1) *realize* the widespread impact of trauma; (2) *recognize* the signs and symptoms of trauma; (3) *respond* by integrating knowledge about trauma into policies, procedures, and practices; and (4) seek to actively *resist* re-traumatization (SAMHSA 2012, 2014). SAMHSA (2014) also outlines six core principles to a trauma-informed approach: (1) safety; (2) trustworthiness and transparency; (3) peer support; (4) collaboration and mutuality; (5) empowerment, voice, and choice; and (6) cultural, historical, and gender issues.

A trauma informed approach has several elements of an asset-based approach. Specifically, it emphasizes capacity and intentionality, focuses on personal relationships, invites meaningful participations, provides opportunities for skill building, concentrates on solutions to the context/systems, recognizes interrelationships, and concentrates on potential solutions. Schools that have implemented a trauma-informed approach have reported increases in student test scores and social mobilization; decreases in emotional dysregulation, psychological distress, and PTSD symptoms; improvements in self-advocacy, coping, confidence, and friendship quality; as well as strengthened relationships between students and school personnel (Fondren et al. 2020; Kataoka et al. 2011; Langley et al. 2015; Mendelson et al. 2015; Santiago et al. 2018; Stein et al. 2003; Wall 2021).

Adverse childhood experiences (ACEs) are potentially traumatic events that occur in childhood and include violence, abuse, and growing up in a family with mental health or substance use problems (CDC 2019). An individual can experience trauma due to an event, series of events, or set of circumstances that is physically or emotionally harmful or life threatening and that has lasting adverse effects on the individual's functioning and mental, physical, social, emotional, or spiritual well-being (Hughes et al. 2017). Not all negative experiences are traumatic, but all traumatic experiences are negative and can have lasting effects (Boullier and Blair 2018).

Unsurprisingly, vulnerable youth, including those who identify as Black, who have interacted with the criminal justice system, and identify as LGBTQ+, are disproportionately impacted by multiple forms of trauma. For example, exposure to at least one ACE is highest among poor youths, with Black youths reporting the highest rates (López et al. 2017). Black youths are also more likely to report multiple ACEs relative to their White counterparts (Bruner 2017; Maguire-Jack et al. 2020; Slopen et al. 2016; Strompolis et al. 2019). One study found that 96 percent of youths who were involved in the criminal justice system had at least one ACE, twice the rate of the general population (Felitti et al. 2019). Another study found that 43 percent of LGBTQ+ youth surveyed experienced four or more ACEs, more than twice the rate of the general population (Craig et al. 2020). Ensuring that schools implement trauma-informed practices may not only enhance academic outcomes of these youths but also support their long-term health and mental health.

Trauma-informed schools seek to create educational environments that are responsive to the needs of trauma-exposed youths through the implementation of effective practices and systems-change strategies (Chafouleas et al. 2016; Overstreet and Chafouleas 2016). Trauma-informed schools implement practices and policies that align with the four Rs described above. For example, multitiered supports that align the goals and principles of trauma-informed schools include supports for student safety, positive interactions, culturally responsive practices, peer supports, targeted supports, and strategies that support the individualized needs of students (Cavanaugh 2016; Walkley and Cox 2013). In addition, universal screenings for trauma exposure can maximize detection of students' exposure to trauma and enable schools to respond to those students with the highest need and ameliorate or prevent negative outcomes (A. Gonzalez et al. 2016). These approaches can also help prevent re-traumatization of students because school personnel can begin to consider trauma as a root cause of behaviors and consider consequences for behaviors that are supportive of students and not punitive (Dorado et al. 2016; Paccione-Dyszlewski 2016; Wall 2021). This shift in perspective may be an essential tool for reducing racial disparities in academic outcomes and suspensions.

Having trauma-focused professional development opportunities for all school personnel (not only teachers) can create a shared understanding of the prevalence of trauma exposure, build consensus for trauma-informed approaches, and foster support for the adoption of system-wide trauma-informed approaches (Overstreet and Chafouleas 2016). Such training often includes providing resources on strategies to create a friendly, warm environment—an environment that both meets the learning needs of students but also provides comfort and security (Wiest-Stevenson and Lee 2016). Despite the racial disparities observed in trauma exposure, there continues to be a dearth of trauma-informed trainings to assist school personnel in their development of the awareness, knowledge, and skills needed to discuss topics of racism-related stress and trauma within the school context (Alvarez 2020; Bernard et al. 2021). Implementing trauma-informed training that is culturally responsive enables all students to see positive representations of their culture in the educational process and can foster increased resilience and cultural pride (Blitz et al. 2016; Goldenberg 2014).

Example of Trauma-Informed Approaches: Restorative Practices in Baltimore City Schools

Restorative practices are a set of strategies used to build social capital and achieve social discipline through participatory learning and decision-making, which enables people to restore and build community (Pennell 2006; Thorsborne and Blood 2013; Zehr 2015). Consistent with a trauma-informed approach, restorative practices (RPs) teach educators to shift from punitive disciplinary practices to approaches that resolve problems. Urban districts like the Baltimore City Public Schools (City Schools) implemented RPs to improve school climate by building meaningful relationships in school communities, reframing school discipline, and supporting student safety, well-being, and success (Eisenberg and Smith 2020). Specifically, City Schools adopted a cohort model to the districtwide implementation of restorative practices. The first cohort consisted of fourteen schools that the district designated as "intensive learning sites" to receive training and coaching in restorative practices beginning in the 2018–19 academic year. Each school in the cohort created an individualized implementation plan in collaboration with City Schools personnel, and Open Society Institute (OSI) funded restorative practitioners, including the Positive Schools Center. Examples of restorative practices included restorative circles, communication techniques (e.g., affective statements and restorative questions), and formal restorative conferences. An evaluation following the implementation found that the use of restorative circles among students was the most common form of RP used. In addition, most schools were able to integrate restorative practices training and lead restorative circles into the school day. Finally, schools that implemented RPs had a 44 percent decrease in suspensions and reported improved school climate and strengthened relationships between students and teachers. A detailed description of RP is provided in chapter 8.

Resilience Building

Although scholars vary their definitions of resiliency, they agree that the theory is one based on strengths rather than deficits (Ungar 2011). Resiliency can be defined as a set of multilevel processes that enable youths to adapt and develop positive well-being in the face of adversity (Van Breda 2001). Resilience is not only an individual construct but one that is relational and present across multiple levels, such as the family, school, and community. Effective resiliency-promoting interventions must address the multiple levels of influences in a young person's life. Resiliency is not static like a trait and is useful when faced with chronic or acute adversity like abuse and neglect, growing up in unsupportive or overly stressed family environments, experiencing poor quality education, and other environmental challenges like poverty and social exclusion. While chronic and acute adversities can overlap, research has shown chronic events to predict poor adult outcomes more reliably (Doll and Lyon 1998). Adversity is necessary for resilience to exist. Specifically, resiliency is observed when youths overcome the negative effects of risk exposure, cope successfully with traumatic experiences, and can reduce or avoid the negative trajectories associated with such risks (Fergus and Zimmerman 2005).

Zimmerman and colleagues suggest that assets and resources serve as promotive factors to ignite resiliency (Fergus and Zimmerman 2005; Zimmerman 2013). Assets are internal qualities such as self-esteem, self-efficacy, problem-solving skills, faith, and optimism. Resources are external factors that allow youths to learn, grow, and practice skills. Examples of resources are parental support, mentors, and extracurricular activities including sports. Assets and resources are embedded in a network of social relationships with families, friends, schools, and communities. This network, or social ecology, creates the conditions under which promotive factors can be accessed (Ungar 2011). Resilience trajectories are heavily influenced by interactions between the family, school, and societal systems (Luthar and Zelazo 2003). Thus, this approach has several elements of an asset based approach. Specifically, it emphasizes capacity and intentionality, attends to the context/systems, recognizes interrelationships, and concentrates on solutions or potential.

There are three reasons that make schools an ideal setting to promote resilience. First, the increasing levels of adverse experiences by youths and their family warrant the need for resilience. Second, schools provide access to large numbers of youths for prolonged periods of time and at critical times of development. Finally, schools often also have the infrastructure and values that are conducive to supporting the development of resilience in young people (Doll and Lyon 1998). Fortunately, schools have continued to use their resources to respond to the ever-changing needs of students.

Resiliency programs in schools range considerably in aim, skills taught, outcomes, and priority population (Dray et al. 2017; Henderson and Milstein 2003; J. J. Liu et al. 2017). Many resiliency programs use cognitive behavioral therapy as an orienting framework, but they also include features such as social and emotional learning, psychological well-being therapy, mindfulness, and the affective-behavioral-cognitive-dynamic (ABCD) model. Cognitive competence, problem-solving/decision-making, cooperation and communication, and coping skills are the most common skills taught through resiliency programs. Often, programs provide strategies both for students and school personnel to create a school environment that is supportive for students facing adversity. Findings from resiliency programs have shown improvements in student resilience and protective factors, including frequency of use of coping skills, internalizing behaviors, and self-efficacy (Fenwick-Smith et al. 2018). They have also shown decreases in depressive symptoms, externalizing behaviors and problems, and general psychological distress (Hodder et al. 2017).

While resiliency programs can focus on the entire school, many have focused on specific subgroups, such as those who are from low-income families or identify as a racial, ethnic, or sexual minority youth. The prevalence of health and mental health risks associated with these subgroups suggest that targeted strategies be developed for them because general programs may not address some of their primary stressors or provide relevant skills that consider their marginalized identities (R. Anderson et al. 2018; Bryan et al. 2020; Craig 2013; Graham-Bermann and Halabu 2004; Heck 2015; Kumi-Yeboah et al. 2021). Youths who face greater adversity require more protective factors to overcome them (Fergus and Zimmerman 2005). Providing resilience-building programs that enhance social justice, facilitate empowerment, and provide opportunities for youths to uncover their strengths work well for marginalized and vulnerable youth (Boyden and Mann 2005; Singh and Salazar 2010). Furthermore, creating a climate that is ripe for resiliency to thrive is critical. Such environments foster caring relationships with others, family engagement, the availability of prosocial role models, and meaningful involvement in their school and community (Bryan et al. 2020, 23).

Example of Resilience Building in Schools: The Aban Aya Youth Project

The Aban Aya Youth Project (AAYP) was developed in Chicago to compare curriculum-based interventions designed to reduce the rate of growth of violence among Black adolescents from grades 5 through 8 (Fagen and Flay 2009; L. C. Liu and Flay 2009; Segawa et al. 2005). Aban Aya is the Ghanaian term for protection (as in fence) and self-determination (endurance and resourcefulness). The interventions include principles that promote Black cultural values such as unity, self-determination, and responsibility, as well as culturally based teaching methods, and inclusion of Black history and literature. Research on the efficacy of AAYP demonstrated that, consistent with other resiliency programs, students who received the social development curriculum—which focused on reducing risky behaviors—learned cognitive-behavioral skills, as well as strategies to build self-esteem and empathy, manage stress and anxiety, develop interpersonal relationships, resist peer pressure, and develop decision-making, problem-solving, conflict resolution, and goal-setting skills. Additionally, males who received a health enhancement curriculum focused on promoting healthy behaviors exhibited lower rates of growth in risk behaviors, including provoking behavior, school delinquency, combined behavior, substance use, and sexual activity.

Critical Youth Engagement

Critical youth engagement (CYE), also known as critical youth empowerment, is the "meaningful participation and sustained involvement of a young person in an activity that has a focus outside himself or herself" and brings their voice into community dialogue (Pancer et al. 2002, 49). Critical youth engagement is situated at the intersection of youth leadership, organizing, and participatory action research (YPAR) (M. Fox et al. 2010). CYE recognizes that young people have knowledge and power, particularly regarding the world they live, attend school, and play in, and the injustices and problems they encounter in those worlds, and it focuses on the critical analysis of those worlds. This means recognizing structural forces like racism, sexism, homophobia, and classism and helping young people understand how these forces work and impact their lives. Lastly, critical analysis is linked to action. Scholars have argued for youth voices in education reform, and students have demanded youth voices at the highest levels of educational administration (Levin 2000); critical youth engagement provides a framework for authentically engaging those voices so that young people are collaborating with adults to address the problems in their schools.

While there are a few different models of critical youth engagement in education (Chinman and Linney 1998), they share six key dimensions, including: (1) a welcoming and safe environment, (2) meaningful participation and engagement, (3) equitable power sharing between youths and adults, (4) engagement in critical reflection on interpersonal and socio-political processes, (5) participation in socio-political processes to effect change, and (6) integrated individual- and community-level empowerment (Jennings et al. 2006). Taken together, these dimensions allow young people to be fully engaged in driving change in education and highlight the components of this approach that align with all asset-based approaches, including a focus on personal relationships, acknowledgment of contribution, an invitation to meaningful participation, and opportunities for skill building or learning.

Critical youth engagement in school settings is particularly necessary for vulnerable youths. Research on youth civic engagement notes that youths who attend urban schools, youths of color, immigrant youths, and young people living in poverty were typically more engaged than their White suburban peers (Flanagan et al. 2007; Lutkus et al. 1999; Sherrod 2005), yet there is little accounting for the opportunities made available to these youths. Conversely, CYE in schools engaging vulnerable youth can raise equity issues that often are minimized by adults. Research suggests that young people and schools benefit from this type of engagement by increasing school bonding and student agency for change (Zeldin et al. 2018; Mitra 2004).

Example of Critical Youth Engagement in Schools: Gender and Sexuality Alliances

Gender and sexuality alliances (previously known as gay–straight alliances [GSAs]) are student-run organizations that bring together LGBTQ+ youth with youth allies, and they work together to build community within the school and organize around issues impacting LGBTQ+ youth in their school. GSAs developed as safe spaces for LGBTQ+ students to support one another (support GSAs) and connect with other LGBTQ+ students and allies (social GSAs). However, many of these student-run clubs are prime examples of CYE in action and have become agents for social change related to racial, gender, and sexual justice in schools (activist GSAs). Research has consistently shown the presence of a GSA in a school, not necessarily individual student participation in the GSA, to significantly impact the school climate for LGBTQ+ youth, even reducing the risk of suicide (Gay, Lesbian & Straight Education Network [GLSEN] 2021; Goodenow et al. 2006).

While GSAs provide opportunities for socializing and providing emotional support for students, the majority focus on helping members address harassment and discrimination in school and working with school staff to create safer school environments. While less common, GSAs also collaborate with other student-led clubs on advocacy or working at the district level to implement LGBTQ+ inclusive policies, including training for school staff (GLSEN 2021). Organizations like the American Civil Liberties Union, Gay Straight Alliance Network, and Gay, Lesbian & Straight Education Network provide resources for students and school staff to support GSAs in middle and high schools, including sample agendas, events, and training materials (GLSEN 2022).

Conclusion

The numbers of underrepresented minority youth experiencing poverty, homelessness, involvement with foster or juvenile care, disconnection from work and school, pregnancy or parenting, or challenges with immigration is significant and growing. Traditionally, behavioral approaches to managing these youths have focused on deficits and emphasized the challenges they face. These approaches are not efficacious. Making a difference will require identifying and implementing asset-based approaches that include a focus on these youths' potential for meaningful contributions, their relationships, and their skills. This chapter has outlined some of those asset-based approaches, documenting the evidence that supports their use in schools.

Schools are essential settings for asset-based approaches to working with adolescents. Schools work with many students and families who come from communities that have endured decades of underinvestment and systemic oppression. Schools have also been subject to this underinvestment and have perpetuated the oppression of students through mechanisms of control rather than opportunities for leadership and growth. Schools have an opportunity to embrace and build asset-based approaches across multiple levels of influence. While asset-based approaches benefit all students, these approaches can be especially important in moving toward optimal health of all youths, including those who may be most vulnerable to negative outcomes and who have been most affected by systemic oppression.

Asset-based approaches like those described in this chapter—positive youth development, trauma-informed approaches, resilience building, and critical youth engagement—share a commitment to focusing on existing strengths and capacity and using resources already available in the communities and schools that serve marginalized and vulnerable youth. They utilize language that is empowering and builds trust with individuals and communities. They acknowledge and leverage resources such as family networks and athletics that can scaffold evidence-based approaches.

Research on these approaches demonstrates that they can be effective—more effective than traditional approaches that have not served marginalized populations in the past. Evidence shows they build resiliency and skill sets that are useful in solving conflicts and raising self-awareness. Rather than seeking to diminish difference, methods like critical youth engagement and restorative practices take on the need for emotional support and strategies for navigating difference and conflict that exist in all communities but disproportionately in schools that enroll large numbers of vulnerable youth. Chapter 8 takes a deeper dive into restorative practices and describes a recent experimental study on its efficacy with adolescents and their families.

5

The Mundane Terror Black Students Experience in Their Schools and Communities

RICHARD LOFTON JR., PHD

> I walk out that door, anything can happen. I'm in the comforts of my own house, I feel comfortable. Once you walk out that door, it's like you are by yourself. It is everywhere. You're out here looking around every day making sure nothing happens to you because you're trying to protect yourself in your school or just walking up and down these streets.
>
> —Leslie, 19

> Don't give us that patronizing rhetoric, we don't need that. We need to change the structural racism in the system. We got to get the drugs off the street. Violence is all around us. We got to get people to get good, stable jobs where they can be able to feed their families. We need to just get rid of these boarded-up homes and develop great businesses of our own. It also takes education. We really need to educate the people who doesn't come from that community to fully understand what we go through on a daily basis. This violence is serious.
>
> —Dion, 21

Leslie and Dion are two Black youths who grew up in West Baltimore and graduated from the Baltimore City Public School System. While reflecting on their educational experiences, they brought up the pervasive violence they encountered while aiming to get to school every day and obtain a diploma. These students did not have the privilege of safe streets surrounding their school or neighborhoods, nor safe school buses that transported them from home to their schools. Leslie and Dion are like many youths who attend a predominantly Black, disinvested school district embedded in high-poverty neighborhoods that lack resources and opportunities (Carter and Welner 2013). As these youths mentioned above, they are not only prone to encountering violence, which is consistent with the social scientific data, but they also suffer from a deepening of precarity (Stovall 2020) when it comes to housing, employment, food security, education, and Black-owned businesses. For them, violence is "everywhere" and "all around us," a mundane part of their everyday lives.

This chapter takes the position that this precarity is not rooted in the actions of Black students but instead is linked to a deeper analysis rooted in anti-Blackness, which has taken the form of structural violence (Rylko-Bauer and Farmer 2016) and positioned Black students to endure suffering in their schools (Dumas 2014, 1–29) and neighborhoods. Latoya Baldwin Clark (2022) suggested that "structural violence occurs in the context of domination, where poor Black children are marginalized and isolated, vulnerable to lifelong subordination across many domains" (p. 499). Rylko-Bauer and Farmer (2016) referred to this structural violence as "the violence of injustice and inequity" (p. 47) that dehumanizes and distributes suffering. Rather than focusing solely on interpersonal violence to address healthy and safe schools, this chapter deviates from a myopic view of personal interactions to discerning how anti-Blackness has taken the form of structural violence and positioned Black youths to undergo suffering, which Hartman (1997) referred to as mundane terror and which I adopt to represent the everyday structural violence that students endure that leads to interpersonal violence, harm, and suffering. In this study, youths reported mundane terror through the everyday disinvestment and unprotection they experience daily in their schools and communities that hinder life opportunities and resources they need to thrive in society (Rylko-Bauer and Farmer 2016).

To explore the mundane terror that youths endure, I performed two main tasks. First, by employing Baltimore as a case study, I reviewed literature that can help readers understand how anti-Blackness through structural violence has positioned poor Black youths to endure mundane terror. While this chapter mainly tells a Baltimore story, this history is connected to a larger American story when it comes to anti-Blackness, racial segregation, and housing. The importance of this review is to move beyond narrow views of poor Black neighborhoods as sites of disorganization and violence (Wacquant 1997). Instead, the literature pointed to structural arrangements through policies and practices that have fostered violence, exclusion, exoticism, and dehumanization, while maintaining Whiteness as property (Harris 1993). Second, I chose to highlight the voices and experiences of thirty-nine Black youths who identified mundane terror in their homes, schools, and communities, as illustrated by the quotes from Leslie and Dion to start this chapter. In the process, the youths' distrust of police protection to prevent them from mundane terror is also highlighted. This review, then, redirects our attention to safe and healthy schools by acknowledging how society has normalized structural violence—persistent harm, violence, and suffering—to position Black youths to endure ongoing mundane terror in their social world.

Conceptualizing Anti-Blackness, Structural Violence, and Mundane Terror

To understand the mundane terror that comes from disinvestment and unprotection, and in some cases the experience of harm, violence, and suffering that youths like Leslie and Dion endure in their schools and neighborhoods, I employed a BlackCrit (Dumas and ross 2016) lens to explore how anti-Blackness has produced structural violence fostering mundane terror (Hartman 1997). ross (2020) referred to anti-Blackness as a "theoretical framework that illuminates society's inability to recognize [Black] humanity—the disdain, disregard and disgust for our existence" (n.p.). Disdain, disregard, and disgust have perpetuated terrorizing experiences for Black Americans since the beginning of American history. Particularly since slavery in the United States, the experiences of terror that Black people have suffered through structural violence have deprived them of justice and equity. Researchers often call attention to interpersonal violence without acknowledging how structural violence has positioned Black people to endure it. Saidiya Hartman (1997) asked researchers and theorists to capture not only "the shocking and the terrible" terrorizing experiences but also the mundane "scenes in which terror can hardly be discerned" (p. 4). To get closer to the terror that can hardly be discerned, I answered Hartman's call by uncovering the mundane terror that has been structured into many predominantly Black schools and neighborhoods. I argue that structural violence continually and purposefully places Black youths in harm's way.

The Structural Violence of Mundane Terror

A century-old tenet is the idea that the ghetto is a "disorganized" social formation that can be analyzed wholly in terms of lack and deficiencies (individual or collective) rather than by positively identifying the principles that underlie its internal order and govern its specific mode of functioning (Wacquant 1997).

When discussing poor Black neighborhoods, Loic Wacquant, a sociologist, suggested that some researchers examine these spaces as being disorganized without carefully connecting structural arrangements to interpersonal interactions. Rather than exoticizing the deficiencies of Black communities, I discern the structural violence of mundane terror through the lens of research conducted on concentrated poverty and education debt (Ladson-Billings 2006).

Concentrated poverty is a term that social scientists and policymakers employ to explore high poverty levels within a neighborhood and the effects of living in these areas when it mainly comes to crime, violence, lack of achievement, and social isolation (Herring 2019; Jargowsky 2013). Aiming to address President Lyndon B. Johnson's 1964 War on Poverty, the US Bureau of the Census started measuring high-poverty neighborhoods in the late 1960s and early 1970s (Herring 2019). Then, in the late 1980s and 1990s, researchers such as William Julius Wilson (1987) brought attention to the measurement of neighborhood poverty and its effects on the neighborhood. Researchers have suggested that concentrated poverty is associated with neighborhood effects, namely more crime, violence, homicides, evictions, psychological distress, and health problems (Sampson et al. 2018; Sharkey 2013; Valdez et al. 2007). Social scientists have often pointed out how neighborhood effects impact educational outcomes, particularly in the areas of absenteeism, standardized test scores, and cognitive abilities (S. Anderson et al. 2014; Chetty et al. 2014; Sharkey and Elwert 2011). According to these researchers, many Black students live in concentrated poverty and encounter neighborhood effects that impede their social mobility (Chetty et al. 2014).

The impact of neighborhood effects in areas of concentrated poverty has been detailed and explored, but what is missing from this research is the analysis of how anti-Blackness and structural violence have made many Black students vulnerable to high-poverty environments by marginalizing and racially quarantining them to endure mundane terror. Reflecting Wacquant's (1997) earlier quote, I conclude that these areas of high poverty are neither disorganized spaces that should be exoticized nor nefarious neighborhood effects; rather, they are linked to structural arrangements that foster and perpetuate mundane terror.

Using Baltimore as an example of this concept of mundane terror, we can discern the anti-Blackness and structural violence that continue today. The problematic history is not necessarily recent; anti-Blackness took the form of structural violence in 1910, when the then-mayor of Baltimore, John Barry Mahool, and other residents had the mentality (Power 1983) that suggested "Blacks should be quarantined in isolated slums in order to reduce the incidence of civil disturbance, to prevent the spread of communicable disease into the nearby White neighborhoods, and to protect property values among the White majority" (Rothstein 2015).

The mayor's sentiment was that Blackness should be quarantined in segregated neighborhoods to reduce disturbance, prevent communicable disease, and protect White property (Harris 1993). Blackness was the disease—the problem—that required quarantining to ensure White people's lives and property were safe. After the mayor's speech, structural violence took the form of racial ordinances (Power 1983), redlining (Pietila 2010), blockbusting (Orser 1994), aggressive urban renewal displacement, subprime lending (Norris 2009; Powell 2009), and the disinvestment of capital and resources in predominantly Black neighborhoods. Researchers have called these predominantly Black neighborhoods in Baltimore the "Black Butterfly" (L. T. Brown 2021), suggesting that these areas form a butterfly shape, while White areas are shaped like an L. By shedding closer light on Mayor Mahool's sentiment in 1910 and the subsequent implemented practices of structural violence, researchers can see how concentrated poverty in Baltimore has always been—and continued to be—linked to a racial quarantine blocking and excluding Blackness from resources, opportunities, employment, and property through a process of dehumanization. In Baltimore, concentrated poverty is a series of person-made decisions that hold Black people back because of White fear of Blackness and its association with violence, crime, and destruction of Whiteness as property. Therefore, social isolation, crime, violence, and unemployment did not just happen, they were structured into our society. Now, many Black students are positioned to be in harm's way in these high-poverty neighborhoods.

Structural violence, as Bandy Lee (2016) described it, "constrains [people] from achieving the quality of life that would have otherwise been possible" (p. 110). Schooling is part of that structural violence when it prevents students from developing the academic skills and social connections they need for career and adult success. While the evidence is clear on the importance of education, Maryland has disinvested in Baltimore schools for many years (Shiller and BMORE Caucus 2019). This disinvestment has limited many opportunities and resources for students in the city. Maryland, like other states throughout the United States, includes in its state constitution an educational clause that uses the language related to a "thorough and efficient educational system." Despite the state constitution, Black students far too often do not receive a "thorough," "efficient," "adequate," and "uniform" educational system. According to Gloria Ladson-Billings (2006), Black students must come to terms with an education debt linked to historical, economic, sociopolitical, and moral components. Historically and currently, many Black students have been or are being confronted with unfunded schools linked to inequitable resource distribution

(Carter and Welner 2013), regardless of their state constitutional rights. Confronted with this education debt, scholars have more recently looked beyond the debt to the suffering that pervades many schools—namely, exploitation, disregard, disdain, unrecognition, exclusion, violence, and mundane racial struggles (Baldridge 2020; Dumas 2014, 2016). Building on this education debt and suffering in school, I explored how structural violence specifically positions Black students to endure disinvestment, harm, and violence.

This literature documents the mundane terror that students have been positioned to endure because of anti-Black policies and practices within the structural violence of exclusion, resource blocking, disinvestment, and education debt in underfunded schools. The remaining sections of this chapter highlight how I captured reports of mundane terror in the experiences of Black youths who identified the everyday terror they experience in their neighborhoods and schools.

Capturing the Poverty of Terror: Methods

After the in-custody death of a twenty-five-year-old Black male, Freddie Gray, was attributed to negligence by Baltimore City police officers, I immediately went into the streets of Baltimore to capture how Black students were making sense of his death. I wanted to uncover the circumstances they confronted in their homes, schools, and communities, which cannot be separated from their educational experiences (Coleman et al. 1966). I designed a case study grounded by interviews with thirty-nine Black youths to understand how the injustices and inequalities they encountered in their high-poverty communities and underfunded school district impacted their education.

This case study was sampled in Baltimore because of the well-documented quantitative data highlighting the neighborhood effects that hinder social mobility (Chetty et al. 2014). More recently, scholars have begun studying Baltimore through the lens of the "Black Butterfly"—a metaphor that speaks to racial segregation and disinvestment in Black neighborhoods in Baltimore (L. T. Brown 2021). The "Black Butterfly," which encompasses many areas in Baltimore where Black students and their parents are in position to confront high levels of crime, violence, homelessness, liquor stores, food deserts, check-cashing and payday lending facilities, and unreliable transportation (L. Brown 2016) and comparative families outside of the "Butterfly." The education debt also continues in Baltimore, with schools within the "Butterfly" reflecting the same disinvestment that plagues the neighborhoods themselves. Several reforms have been attempted within the school district over the last twenty years, but researchers have pointed to underfunded school resources as the reason for their failures. Not surprisingly, given the education debt, student test scores since the 1980s have been below state and national averages (Orr 1999; Smerdon and Cohen 2009; Stringfield and Yakimowski-Srebnick 2005). Moreover, many students graduate without the required skills for college and career readiness. According to the Baltimore Education Research Consortium (Baltimore's Promise 2018), of 4,280 graduates of the class of 2009, 26 percent did not enroll in college or join the Maryland workforce six years after graduating, and only 29 percent enrolled in a four-year college.

Findings of Mundane Terror

The youths I interviewed endured the effects of structural violence in two ways. First, they associated the effects of structural violence through segregated and disinvested neighborhoods and schools, which excluded them from the prerequisite resources and social environments that promote healthy and safe places to "actually live." Without academic skills, certified trades, and livable wages, the youths felt everyday terror as they aimed to survive in neighborhoods of high crime, violence, and unemployment. Also, instead of viewing police officers as social actors who want to support and protect their lives, the youths viewed them as the enforcers of structural violence who made them feel like they were prisoners in their community and school.

The Terror of Disinvestment

Schools are intended to be sites where students develop skills to empower and protect themselves to compete and engage actively in a global economy.

Some of these skills are directed toward empowering students toward adult and career success and equipping them with educational "armor" to survive and thrive. In the United States, we often suggest that schools can be the great equalizer. But what if a student lives in a city and attends a school district where very few obtain livable-wage jobs after graduating from high school and college? What if a student attends a school district where city employers often hire out-of-state people instead of workers from the local school district? While schooling is often viewed as the great equalizer, Black students in Baltimore did not find equality, justice, or upward mobility in their educational experiences; rather, they spoke candidly about disinvestment. Schools were viewed as sites of disinvestment that withheld resources, protection, supportive environments, and social connections to develop employment skills.

The following four quotes speak to how disinvestment was associated with not "actually living" and receiving only limited opportunities:

> Like I said, poverty is essentially the lack of opportunity in education, the opportunity to actually live. Especially now. (Ben, age 22)

> City schools are nowhere near on par with county schools. No opportunities. I would say that. Not only education, but social education as well. (Lisa, age 18)

> Education is lacking, nonexistent. That's pretty much. It kills your dreams. (Natasha, age 18)

> We didn't have computer labs. We didn't have enough books, desks, chairs, classrooms, teachers, to be able to teach us. Those are the resources that were basically being taken out. (Alisha, age 21)

In these above quotes, Ben, Lisa, Natasha, and Alisha discussed how their schooling experiences were fraught with disinvestment. Disinvestment in their schooling process stunts their opportunities, dreams, and resources. The students in these interviews did not use conceptualizing terms like social death and mundane terror; their words were more to the point. They wanted the opportunity to "actually live," rather than have "no opportunities," be perceived or valued as "nonexistent," or be consistently confronted with a "lack of resources." Schooling was not an opportunity to live fully in society; it was instead associated with structural violence in the form of disinvestment. As this section continues, these four quotes will continue to be highlighted and connected to these youths' personal stories.

In the first quote, Ben discussed how disinvestment in his high school and neighborhood prevented him from living fully. Two years ago, he lost his father. He graduated from high school five years ago and spent time at a junior college. Aiming to take care of himself, he stopped attending his community college and took on two jobs. He still feels he is confronted with individual and neighborhood poverty with both jobs, for which he works many hours but still has financial issues. In his interview, Ben reflected on how the disinvested educational structure did not offer him Advanced Placement or Honors courses, certified training, or classes teaching financial literacy. While he did graduate from school, the disinvested schooling process did not provide him with opportunities to "actually live."

Ben pointed out that today, to live requires students to be part of a schooling process that invests in their potential. Ben's insight can help researchers and policymakers understand that students can graduate from the schooling process without developing the skills that lead them to become actively alive in a social economy. For Ben and other youths, education is associated with poverty and death; in other words, social death continues in their lives because they are part of a schooling structure that does not prepare them to secure middle-class jobs. Youths felt that they were part of a schooling structure that did not allow them the chance to escape poverty, marginalization, and violence because of the district's disinvestment. While many of these youths at an early age were taught that attending school and graduating would help them with upward social mobility, Ben argued that the schooling process is not the site for it; rather, he felt it is a site of poverty and lack of opportunities leading to a social death.

Disinvestment also took the form of Black youths witnessing how their schools did not look the same or have the same resources as predominantly

White middle-class school districts in the state. Lisa identifies this disinvestment by arguing that the Baltimore City Public School System is not on "par" with other school districts in the state. She associated the education system she attended with a place with "no opportunities." She further suggested that educational structure did not allow for social education. The question, then, remains: What is social education for Lisa? After I posed this question, she responded, "Things that you do outside of class"—that is, social education is work that is not necessarily done in the classroom but through interactions that support youths in developing both academic and social skills. To clarify, she discussed how her schooling process did not help her to gain access to academic clubs, extracurricular activities, or events that supported social connections in school. Also, the school climate for her was not "the best place to learn." Through such comments, Lisa helps researchers understand that disinvestment in educational structures not only hinders access to tangible resources but also more intangible ones such as school climate, extracurricular activities, and social events. Lisa's thinking connects to the body of research suggesting that social connection is vital to youths who are confronted with neighborhood poverty.

While Lisa mentioned intangible factors, other youths witnessed the structural violence of inequity in terms of the lack of resources that block safe and healthy educational experiences. The two main tangible differences that youths reported were the lack of school buses and ineffective school infrastructure. The Baltimore City Public School District is the only one in Maryland that does not supply school buses for their middle and high schoolers—another example of how youths in this school district are positioned to encounter unsafe routes to and from school. Without investment in school buses, the youths acknowledged they are confronted with sexual harassment, fights, arguments with adults, overcrowded situations, homelessness, individuals under the influence of drugs, angry and rude bus drivers, and late buses. The youths showed that the structural arrangement that cannot offer public transportation for middle and high school students positions them to endure unnecessary harm and violence.

In addition, the youths reported poor school conditions that created an unsafe and unhealthy educational environment. Maryland's State Commission Board is assigned to examine all schools. In its evaluation, the board evaluated Baltimore City as above average. The Black youths I interviewed shared that they were forced to miss many days because of extreme temperatures in the building. If they did attend, they were exposed to unhealthy hot and cold conditions in the classroom—a form of mundane terror that they cannot avoid except to lose valuable days. The district's lack of investment in school buses and school infrastructure were two issues that the youths continued to raise that endangered them in what should be a safe environment.

The Black youths also associated disinvestment with killing creativity and dreams. For example, Natasha suggested that the schooling process kills dreams because the lack of resources cannot support the ability to dream and makes it almost nonexistent. Natasha felt the school structure was dead because it does not develop youths for futures of success. While many Americans view the schooling process as supportive of life and ingenuity, Natasha agreed with most of the Black youths who reflected that their educational experiences could snuff out their dreams. According to Alisha, the disinvestment was so bad that many students had no computers, desks, chairs, and books; beyond supplies, their teachers were poorly qualified to develop students' skills for academic success.

The Black youths in this study were aware that society often looks at schooling as the process of developing skills for successful futures, but they regarded the schooling process as maintaining and policing the boundaries of mundane terror. For them, it was almost as if the district's "investment" was not in necessary tools and resources but rather a purposeful investment in not investing in the needed sources of economic success and safety in schools and communities. The youths' statements attested to the reality that they encountered mundane terror through the myriad "lacks" that they could enumerate: resources, opportunities, certified trades, employment, livable wages, and safe school climates. Without positive investments, the students felt socially dead. Not only are the Black youths in Baltimore faced with the mundane terror of no educational structure that supports successful careers and college readiness, but even if they did develop these vital skills, many Black leaders have suggested that these employers are simply not hiring Black youths, even if they graduate. One Black city council member I spoke to made it plain; when asked what we needed to do to change educational experiences and outcomes, he stated:

> We need to increase the number of jobs in Baltimore City for Baltimore City residents and hopefully this is not added on, but you know, develop ways to properly prepare our residents for those jobs. If I could bring twenty thousand manufacturing jobs to Baltimore City, that's what I would do. That would drastically change our city. Right now, the number one industry is drugs, and the number one problem is drugs.

This city council member called attention to Baltimore's lack of employment and industry for Black residents. The youths basically agreed with the city council member when thinking how students are ill equipped because of disinvestment and do not have employers in the city who will hire them. As manifestations of the mundane terror that surfaces through these experiences, many of the Black youths felt they could not live fully, could not dream, could not find social connections or resources that would mold their futures as successful adults. Bypassed and dehumanized in school, the community, and the work world, these youths knew well the existence of mundane terror, whether they named it as such or not. It would continue to impact their lives adversely if it was permitted to thrive in the social infrastructure.

Prisoner in My Community

The Black youths in this study also reported social death as part of the mundane terror caused by police abuse. While many students throughout the United States theoretically associate police officers with the goals of protecting and serving them, the Black youths in Baltimore did not share this view. Instead, the police are instruments by which mundane terror is maintained and reinforced through harm, brutality, and fear. The youths I spoke to live with a consistent fear that the police saw them as the enemy. As a result, regardless of the police officer's race, the youths reported experiencing distrust, brutality, corruption, and disdain from authorities who are supposed to protect and serve all members of the community.

Distrust and brutality were the two most consistent concerns that the youths expressed in their interviews. For example, Kate made this point:

> I know there definitely . . . there's 100 percent of distrust with police. One hundred percent of Black people here do not trust them. But I myself am also a person who I get nervous when my brother or boyfriend is out driving. I've been in the car with a boyfriend, and he was literally pulled over for not having a seat belt on, and he in fact had his seat belt on and was ticketed and had all these issues. I've watched a boyfriend be beaten by the cops just for asking a question. I feel like a lot of police, they get into that mindset of the trouble that's in Baltimore, the knuckleheads, and start to approach everybody that way. Not everybody out here is a criminal.

Kate graduated from the Baltimore City Public School System and was finishing her BA at Morgan State University. She overcame many obstacles to become an educator. What she could not overcome, however, was the distrust and consistent nervousness she felt when thinking about her brother or boyfriend driving. Kate's words zero in on the distrust that Black youths have of police. Not only is there distrust of police but also a social and emotional toll that Black youths face because of corruption and police brutality. In several interviews, the youths discussed newspaper headlines that called out corruption in the city. Moreover, they discussed the police brutality that has killed youths like Freddie Gray in Baltimore or countless other Black individuals across the nation. Many of the youths interviewed discussed this form of mundane terror: the constant fear that police officers will impose their power and control to hurt them without being held accountable for their wrongdoing.

The fear of police brutality is not new to Black people. What is often not discussed is the historical relationship that Black people in Baltimore encountered with policing. According to Adam Malka, policing in Baltimore was developed to control free Black people and prevent them from gaining property and jobs (Malka 2018). Further, Malka pointed out that White mobs and police worked together in the early 1900s to ensure that, as one youth stated, "Blacks stay in their place." More recently, the War on Drugs continues to terrorize Black communities in Baltimore. In this war, Black males on the streets are viewed as the main perpetuators rather than as social actors who have brought drugs into the country. When examining the recommendation to have more police in schools, researchers, policymakers, and educators must understand that many within the Black community believe that police have been historically positioned to control and prevent Black people from living fully and gaining economic freedom.

In addition to social control by the police, the youths perceived that these officers had disdain and disregard for their lives, regardless of the officer's race. Tony illustrated this point:

> I don't know. I don't know why they hate me or if they hate some statistic that they read about people that look like me, so then they're afraid of me, and so then they might do things that are outrageous. I have no idea what it is. I don't know, because some people get off on the fact that they have power of people. I have no idea. I'm so confused about why it is the way it is.

Tony used the word "hate"—a word that was commonly found in my interviews. The youths reported that the police viewed them as "criminals," "low-lifes," "thugs," and "just plain out dirty"; they could not use positive descriptors such as students, citizens, and taxpayers. Tony felt that this myopic view of Blackness was because of bad statistics and stereotypes that people read into Black people. For him, this continues a narrative of Black people as wrongdoers and perpetuates fear that fuels outrageous acts of police brutality. Tony further stated that he has no clear idea why police hate Black people, but the feeling of certain hatred is real. Tony then stated that some police use their power to control Black people. These words clearly illustrate that the youths perceived police officers in their schools and communities as being disdainful and dismissive of their culture, history, and experiences that have been forcibly linked to structural violence.

To avoid potentially fatal encounters with police on the streets of Baltimore, many youths ensure their safety by simply staying at home. Many questions remain regarding the agency of youths and parents in these environments of terror. For the youths, one way to be protected is to stay at home and develop homeplaces where they can humanize and defend themselves from the toxicity of structural violence. For example, Danielle vividly described how she spent most of her time in her house because of the violence:

> Oh no, I did not go outside and play. My mother did not allow me to go outside. Me and brother we had to stay in the house.
>
> It was not safe out there. We watched the news all the time where things happen to people. When we left school, we came home. We did not go anywhere after that.
>
> We never knew what might happen. We were scared that something might happen. So, we just stayed in the house.

Danielle's words connected with many of the young participants. Very few said they played outside with friends or ran up and down the streets of Baltimore. These youths were prevented from accessing opportunities to benefit from recreational parks, enrichment programs, and extracurricular activities that many peers in surrounding districts and well-invested communities take for granted. When they did leave home to participate in activities, some were constantly afraid of the gratuitous violence that may erupt. Parents often demanded they not leave home by themselves. When possible, parents would accompany them or ask their older son to accompany a younger sister in the street. Danielle's comments echoed the inevitable sense that this fear, which confined them to their homes, also created a prison. Missing out on healthy leisure activities, beautiful nature, and camaraderie with friends and family, the Black youths in Baltimore are shortchanged of opportunities to thrive in all circles of their lives: home, school, neighborhood, community. The fear and terror of crime and danger restricted them from living a whole life and moved them toward a slow social death.

Conclusion

While all the chapters in this book examine how to support healthy and safe schools, this chapter brings unique insight by highlighting the social position of Blackness, specifically among Black youths in Baltimore, through the prism of structural violence. I ask researchers, policymakers, and educators to move beyond the idea that Black youths are wrongdoers and examine instead how disinvested communities and underfunded schools continue to perpetuate structural violence as implicit ways to hinder required resources and opportunities needed for social mobility. Through an anti-Black lens, one can identify society's inability to recognize the full citizenship and humanity of all Black people. Even with constitutional provisions in place, there is no investment in guaranteeing that their fundamental human needs and rights will be met. Structural violence has taken the form of disinvestment within predominantly Black schools, which causes students to be deprived of educational skills for academic and career success. Black youths and Black politicians admitted feeling that even if they did develop academic skills, employers would not hire Black students who grew up and attended the Baltimore City Public School System.

The students in this study have described experiencing persistent patterns of scarce resources, fear and danger, and lack of protection and encouragement. More mundane terrors have taken the form of scarcities to survive and thrive physically and academically—or, as Ben summed up, "to actually live." Terror is based on the anti-Black ideology that expects students to develop skills without society's willingness to provide support to address their educational needs and promote college and career readiness. This social inability to humanize the lived experiences of Black students at one point provided the rhetoric of schools as the "great equalizer," but, in fact, the reality is that of a great and inequitable divider.

Poverty is socially constructed. It is a mechanism used to prevent educational opportunities for Black students while also underscoring terrorizing experiences fueled by violence. Black youths constantly fear dangers and, thus, do not have the privilege of focusing only on academic growth. Violence forces them to think consistently about protecting themselves from harm—the harm that comes from struggling to survive in an anti-Black society or confronting hostile authority figures who see Black youths as enemies. When examining the health and safety of schools, we must consider the anti-Black structural violence that has normalized disinvestment and underfunding. In addition, we must ensure that school resources and opportunities will nurture students to live freely and develop necessary skills for academic and economic success. In doing this deep reflection and research, we can convert structural violence and social death into equal opportunities and full lives for all Black students.

Part II

APPROACHES FOR SAFE AND HEALTHY SCHOOLS

6

Schools as Part of a Carceral Ecosystem

ODIS JOHNSON JR., PHD

The national conversation about racialized police violence has ignited debate about the presence of police in the nation's schools and the disproportionate criminalization of minoritized youths. While these conversations are often framed with the goal of achieving safe and healthy schools, in other arenas they are framed by the "school-to-prison" (STP) pipeline concept, which typified the fear that school experiences were leading students to jail cells instead of successful futures. However, some may view the explicit connection of the STP pipeline a bit reductionist and as precluding the exploration of the full range of mechanisms and far-reaching consequences of carceral education.

Using an interest in the nation's desire for safe and healthy schools as the point of departure, this chapter provides a framework for understanding how social control gives rise to carceral education and an ecosystem including the STP pipeline that poses barriers to the health and well-being of youths—especially those from minoritized communities. In doing so, the chapter demonstrates how schools, in recent decades, have undergone their own conversion from schools to prison-like institutions that jeopardize the health and well-being of minoritized youths. Next, the chapter identifies and summarizes seven domains that collude with social control to give rise to carceral education and form a carceral ecosystem of disparity-producing racial health risks. The discussion concludes with recommendations that policymakers, practitioners, researchers, and activists can undertake to dismantle the structures and systems that form the ecosystem of risk and put in its place one of care and well-being.

Establishing a Framework: Social Control, Carceral Education, and the STP Pipeline

Social Control in Relation to Education

The concept of social control concerns how a society maintains social order. Social control is often accomplished via "internal group regulation" (Kirk 2009) in which individuals adhere to and internalize shared norms (Durkheim et al. 1961). Others have noted social control acts as a "repressive moral code" (Massey 1996) in which shame, stigma, and the fear of ostracism leads individuals to conform to social norms. However, as Janowitz (1975) observed, "any social order, including a society with a relatively effective system of social control, will require an element of coercion" (p. 84), or what we call formal social control. Formal social control has been described as the actions of state apparatuses (Althusser 1969) and their technologies (Foucault 1975) that establish the institutional regulation of life (Lacombe 1996), and the laws, government action, and institutions that arise in reaction to perceived deviance (Parsons 1937). It follows that schools are agents of formal social control since most of them are state institutions, or regulated by the state, and because attending them is compulsory, with few allowable exceptions. In schools, social control takes on a few widely acknowledged purposes. These include the maintenance of a safe and orderly environment conducive to learning, socialization of youths through schools' mission to provide character and moral development, and its social function of sorting and allocating individuals into adult roles for the purposes of reproducing the initial expression of social order in the United States—that is, settler colonialism, patriarchy, cisgender domination, and White racial supremacy, among other status hierarchies. In sum, social control is needed to maintain social order, particularly for those in power, and a system of beliefs that forms the edifice of carceral education.

Carceral Education and Student Health

"Carceral" (i.e., of, relating to, or suggesting a jail or prison) education can be understood as the institutional conditions and relationships that over-emphasize the maintenance of order and control, regimented learning, conformity and obedience of students, and its primary device, punishment. Unlike the school-to-prison (STP) pipeline, carceral education extends far beyond the incarceration risks and outcomes youths experience to include an array of social and behavioral outcomes. Carceral education can be viewed as the flip side of school safety, with the same features designed to keep children safe often causing them to feel like suspects and to view their peers as potential threats (Johnson et al. 2019). In this chapter, I argue that carceral education comprises a constellation of interacting, overlapping, and systematically related phenomena that form an ecosystem of risk with serious implications for not only students' educational success but also their health and well-being.

Linkages between carcerality and health in the educational experiences of youths manifest in a few ways. The sense of unfairness students may develop within carceral schools could impact their socio-emotional well-being, including their sense of belonging, self-esteem, and self-concept (R. Bailey et al. 2019; Hirschi 2001). In addition, schools become sites of risk when they emphasize surveillance and policing, potentially leading to prolonged heightened vigilance, which has been indicated in research by the elevated cortisol levels of women of color in high-risk environments (M. Lee et al. 2021). With the "fight or flight" state of mind being reflected in cortisol levels, students may be primed to respond to uncomfortable situations in ways that cause school disruptions, violence, and socio-emotional distress in other students. Unfortunately, schools are most likely to address these coping mechanisms with greater punishment rather than trauma-informed care, or restorative practices as discussed in chapter 9 of this volume (Grant, Douglas, et al. 2022). This cycle sets in motion a self-fulfilling prophecy (A. Ferguson 2001) in which carceral conditions instigate coping mechanisms that, once manifest, are punished by those same carceral conditions, leading to re-traumatization for students (Wade and Ortiz 2017) and heightened criminalization (Mittleman 2018a). This suggests public health researchers and school professionals should consider the carceral character of schools a social determinant of students' mental health.

Others have observed that health services within punitive-oriented schools are often coopted to further the carceral agenda of schools. This has given rise to concerns about "medicated social control" or "pharmacological control" (Moody 2016; Skiba, Michael, et al. 2002) in which children are identified as having behavioral disorders and subsequently prescribed medication to control their hyperactivity and related disorders. While such diagnoses are useful for some children who receive them (C. Kim et al. 2010), there is concern about the disproportionately higher rate of identification of minoritized youths for medication and the racialized school processes that lead to these identification disparities (Skiba, Michael, et al. 2002). Future studies are needed to explore whether significant linkages between the carceral structure of schools and rates of hyperactivity treatment for Black students remain after considering schools' average levels of disorder and urban location.

Equally troubling and closely related to rates of hyperactivity disorder are racial inequities in students' identification for special educational services and removal from mainstream classrooms (Skiba, Michael, et al. 2002). Disproportionate and excessive special education identification frames the practice as another track of social control within carceral institutions, with the overrepresentation of minoritized youths as a conspicuous indicator. Instead of leading to less punitive or more accommodating responses to perceived misbehavior for all students with special needs, a student's identification as such seems to have the opposite effect when they are Black. For example, Black students with disabilities lost approximately seventy-seven more days of instruction due to suspensions compared to White students with disabilities (United States Commission on Civil Rights 2019). These racially disparate patterns arising from carceral education give life to what the American Psychological Association recognizes as racial stress (2018) and other researchers identify as racial trauma

(R. Carter et al. 2017). The racial disparities produced in strict school communities are associated with a host of other stressors, from feelings of helplessness and surrender when directly or vicariously confronted with racial barriers (Brunson and Miller 2006), to feelings of isolation and perceived fraudulence (i.e., imposter syndrome) for those who experience success despite racial barriers (Bernard et al. 2018; McGee et al. 2021). These are but a few of the ways in which carceral education is related to health.

How the STP Pipeline Differs from Social Control and Carceral Education

While carceral education constitutes the structures of social control, the school-to-prison pipeline serves as one of carceral education's concretized systems of student sorting and allocation into postsecondary social positions. While often referred to as a "metaphor," the STP pipeline has evolved alongside mass incarceration (Alexander 2010; Fasching-Varner et al. 2014) into an identifiable mechanism with a growing frequency of occurrence in the lives of school-age individuals. For example, data reveal that between 2005 and 2014, law enforcement in San Bernardino, California, arrested 6,923 minors on the streets but over 30,000 while serving schools (Ferriss 2015), intimating the criminal referral system of many school districts is as robust as many other educational tracks, making the STP pipeline more than just a metaphor.

Racial disproportionalities in the rate at which youths are referred to law enforcement are blatant and suggest schools—and the law enforcement within them—take harsher approaches to handling the behavior of students of color. For example, state-mandated reporting of "disproportionate minority contact" (DMC) rates in Maryland show that, in Prince George's County, Black and Hispanic youths between the ages of ten and eighteen were referred to juvenile intake at a rate 2.40 and 1.87 times that of Whites who had committed similar offenses, respectively (Young et al. 2011). More recent numbers show that these DMC rates for Maryland's Black youths are still large, standing at 2.39, 2.26, and 2.42 times higher than that of Whites for secured detention, time served in juvenile corrections, and transfer to adult court, respectively (Governor's Office of Crime

Control and Prevention 2019). These DMC rates are not limited to the state of Maryland but are pervasive enough to prompt the United Nations (UN) to register its concern about the existence of a "school-to-prison pipeline" for Black children in the United States (United Nations Human Rights 2016).

Yet the "school to prison" phrase does have metaphorical value beyond its reference to an apparent educational pathway to incarceration. In addition to being a conduit of social and material relations that transitions students from classrooms to jail cells, "school to prison" may most appropriately refer to the recent transformation of school itself into prison-like institutions. The evidence reviewed later in this chapter will show that, in recent decades, schools have witnessed increases in the use and introduction of advanced surveillance technologies, more numerous statutes with stiffer penalties for perceived student misbehavior, and a greater presence of armed law enforcement. Therefore, researchers and policymakers should be concerned with how schools are transitioning from "schools to prisons" as much as they are about how youths "transition from schools to prisons."

STP in Relation to Student Health and Well-Being

Many of the same health risks related to carceral education apply to the school-to-prison pipeline. However, interaction with police and penal systems may exacerbate these health risks and produce additional ones. Unfortunately, available data do not make this connection very clear for several reasons. First, police encounters with school-age youths are often considered "pedestrian stops" (especially those near or on school campus grounds) and laws in most jurisdictions do not require officers to log pedestrian encounters (Policing Project 2019). With the number of pedestrian stops missing from the total number of youth and officer encounters, the estimation of the likelihood of any police-related health outcome remains challenging. Second, officers often use force to restrain suspects, yet data about whether students sustained injuries due to officers' use of force is largely uncollected or is revealed only if video is publicly released or criminal or civil charges are filed. Third, while many state statutes have made causing emotional distress in school (i.e., bullying) a felony with risks of imprisonment (Matos 2017), the profiling, physical restraining, intimidation, provocation, humiliation, and verbal assault youths receive from officers is considered within the officers' line of duty, even when it is not an appropriate response to normative child and adolescent behavior. Nonetheless, the frequent appearance of video footage in social media outlets showing officers use excessive force on youths of color in schools suggests such data should be collected, along with data about the mental health implications for youths who are greeted at school doors, every day, by security they may suspect are perpetrators of similar abuses. Carceral education normalizes, legitimizes, and makes mundane the trauma students experience by building terror into their daily routines (see chapter 5 in this volume).

The Carceral Ecosystem of Social Determinants and Risks

Social control is pursued in social life with the assistance of many other structural and systemic forces to establish carceral education and subsequently, the social reproduction of White settler, cisgender, heteronormative, and patriarchal dominance—the initial expression of social order in the United States. Within the domain of social control, punishment, culture, law, neighborhoods, political economy, technologies, and law enforcement serve an important role in enabling formal social control. These seven overlapping, interrelating, and mutually reinforcing components form a carceral ecosystem in support of social control, in which carceral education takes shape to concretize tracks, pipelines, programs, and opportunities that impact student health. In the sections that follow, I provide a brief overview of each of these important domains.

Political Economic Neoliberalism

Political economic neoliberalism supports the application of market principles to social objectives and problems, while purporting to decentralize government control over social services and increasing individual freedom of choice (D. Harvey 2007; Lipman 2011). The view of schools as the primary contexts of labor market skill development (Bowles and Gintis 1976), and as particularly difficult to reform agents of adult role allocation within society's economic apparatus (Henig et al. 2001), has set the stage for policymakers and economists to promote market approaches to educational change. Yet, decentralization and the introduction of market principles has also advanced carceral education, namely through the expansion of "no excuses" charter schools.

Charter schools reflect the decentralization of public education because they are released from the zoned local attendance requirements that traditional public schools have, adopt different approaches to learning and discipline, and market those approaches to compete for students from families that have a choice in which school their child attends (Lipman 2011). No-excuses charter schools are a subgroup of charter schools that typically have, among other features, a highly regimented educational experience, and expansive zero-tolerance policies that include penalties for minor infractions and personal movement (e.g., position of hands, walking with hands at side) (Golann 2015; Advocates for Children 2015). Consequently, charter schools tend to have inordinately high suspension rates, like in New York City, where charter schools enrolled roughly 7 percent of the district's student population, but levied nearly 42 percent of its suspensions in 2014 (Joseph and CityLab 2016). Investment in exclusionary disciplinary practices in no-excuses charter schools like KIPP (Knowledge Is Power Program) have led to high student attrition, in some schools reaching 50 percent, undoubtedly positively inflating the network's student test outcomes through selectively pushing out targeted students (Woodworth 2008; Henig 2008).

Studies have touted the potential of no-excuses charter schools without any thought to how their strict disciplinary approaches possibly impacted attrition in the estimation of charter lottery effects on learning (see examples at Cohodes 2018; Gleason et al. 2010). The focus on academic measures in these studies in defining school "quality" and as the singular reason to call for expansion of no-excuses charters minimizes the troubling rate of pushouts from charter schools (Advocates for Children 2015) and how they impact students' dispositions toward learning (Golann 2015), mental health (R. Bailey et al. 2019), and risks of incarceration (Mittleman 2018a).

While it may appear that decentralization relaxes state regulation of schooling, in no-excuses charters it has the perverse effect of strengthening state surveillance and penalties for the individual freedoms of movement and gesture that were previously taken for granted. Within a political economic perspective, the implementation of militaristic behavioral routines and expectations of thoughtless compliance represents the transformation of schools from what Althusser (1969) called society's primary ideological state apparatuses (ISAs) to more repressive state apparatuses (RSAs), a term Althusser reserved for the courts, military, and police. Mirroring the "school-to-prison" transformation, the repurposing of schools from ISAs to RSAs via charters has been enacted with minoritized youths in mind. Currently, charter schools disproportionately serve minoritized students, constituting 25 and 34 percent of total enrollment for Black and Hispanic students in 2018, respectively (National Center for Education Statistics 2018a). As Eva Moskowitz, the CEO of Success Academy, one of New York City's largest charter networks, commented about the largely Black parents with kids in her schools, they "believe in stricter discipline" (Golann and Debs 2019).

Statutory and Policy Context

The statutory and policy context of carceral education consists of numerous laws at the federal, state, and local level; their enforcement; and the severity of the consequence for perceived offenders. While a review of all laws that contribute to carceral conditions in school is not possible in this chapter, this section reviews zero tolerance, disturbance laws, and changing state statutes to illustrate the role of federal law, stiffer state penalties, and subjective enforcement at the local levels in furthering carceral education. Considering zero tolerance first, the Gun-Free Schools Act of 1994 ushered in the era of zero tolerance, urging states that received federal funds to enact inflexible and mandatory triggers for expulsion for students who were suspected of safety violations (United States Congress 1993; Skiba and Rousch 2006). These mandatory triggers were not limited to students in possession of weapons, but they were also extended to fighting, physical contact or assault against school personnel, and other violations. While these policy positions seem reasonable, they had the effect of removing the consideration of intent in adjudicating perceived misconduct and circumventing due process protections for youths. Under these laws, the reason for the offense did not matter, and school actors who knew the children involved and the circumstances of the incident best could do nothing to stop expulsions.

As zero tolerance became widespread, states also reclassified what would otherwise be normative child and adolescent behavior into prosecutorial offenses. In 2017, for instance, a Missouri state law went into effect reclassifying fighting and causing emotional distress from misdemeanor offenses to class A felonies, punishable with up to four years in jail for age groups as young as 7 (Matos 2017). Missouri's law is another example of how more severe responses to perceived deviance have facilitated the school-to-prison transformation of schools.

Finally, school disturbance and disruption laws have been adopted in at least twenty-two states as of 2017, encompassed by many other states' disorderly conduct and disturbing the peace statutes (Rivera-Calderón 2017). Inasmuch as zero tolerance lacks flexibility and undermines the agency of school leaders to apply punishments that fit the circumstances of safety violations, school disturbance and disruption laws rely on subjective assessments of what constitutes a disturbance and are therefore susceptible to implicit and conscious bias, and racial injustice when discretion and leniency are not extended equally to all students. Revisiting the previously mentioned rate of minor arrests in San Bernardino, roughly a third (i.e., 9,900) of them were for "disturbing the peace," which could include any action that distracts a teacher. These numbers have raised questions about whether "most of these arrests were necessary for public safety" (Ferriss 2015) and to what extent these perceived norm violations interfere with the learning of students' peers.

Cultural Policing

Schools have long maintained a commitment to moral and character education (H. Mann 1952) in addition to their role of reproducing the distribution of society's knowledge from one generation to the next (Bourdieu 1977). In most schools, this commitment to have students reflect the morals and character of dominant social classes is enshrined in district policies and state statutes. A school's dress code is an example of this, reflecting the institution's preference for student apparel and hairstyle, among other cultural aesthetics, and giving school personnel the authority to apply sanctions to perceived deviations from preferred social norms. While healthy and affirming schools often have dress codes in place to minimize possible distractions in the classroom, carceral education's commitment to cultural policing uses dress codes to punish student departures from dominant cultural tastes and aesthetics. The cases of Andrew Johnson and DeAndre Arnold stand as examples; both Black students were barred from school activities, and in the case of the latter, suspended, until they agreed to cut their dreadlocks (Ahmed 2018; Griffith 2020).

Schools claim that the young men's hair length, not cultural style, were the reasons why they were punished (Griffith 2020). Implicit within this admission is the schools' preference for normative gender appearances, that is, boys and young men with short hair. Cultural policing of students' gender and sexual orientation expression occurs routinely, leaving them (especially gender nonconforming girls) with a greater likelihood of receiving harsh discipline roughly three times that of their heterosexual counterparts (Himmelstein and Brückner 2011). This increases students' emotional and mental distress and vulnerability to similar attacks from peers (Hunt and Moodie-Mills 2012).

Cultural policing is also fueled by adultification, or the bias (whether implicit or conscious) that causes school personnel to view youths of color as older than they are, less innocent, and more threatening and lascivious (Epstein et al. 2017). Through the lens of adultification, the stylistic expression of Black girls is often viewed as "unlady-like" (Ibrahim et al. 2021), and the youthful behavior of Black preschool-age kids deserving of severe punishments. The US Office of Civil Rights reports that Black children made up roughly 18.2 percent of preschool enrollment in 2017, but 43.3 percent of those suspended and 38.2 percent of those expelled (Office for Civil Rights 2021). In sum, cultural policing is a practice of meting out sanctions for perceived deviations from normative standards of cultural expression and bias in discerning age-appropriate behavior along several dimensions of identity, including gender, sexual orientation, and race, among others.

Technologies

Technologies are indispensable to the carceral ecosystem because social control relies on systems of surveillance to detect perceived deviance, encourage self-regulation, and restrict liberties (Foucault 1975). While technologies of social control in the Focauldian sense would include any technique of domination, this chapter considers electronic technologies of search and surveillance. On this dimension, the School Survey on Crime and Safety reveals that between 1999 and 2008 growth in schools' surveillance methods was shared by all schools (Addington 2014). Nonetheless, recent work from the Race, Gender, and Social Control in STEM Lab at the Center for Safe & Healthy Schools at Johns Hopkins University estimates four times as many Black students attended high schools heavily reliant on surveillance technologies than attended the least reliant schools. Schools that used surveillance heavily had elevated suspension rates, lowered math scores, and lowered rates of college entry (Johnson and Jabbari 2021). No data exists about the capacity of these schools to meet the mental health needs of students who cope with the weight of surveillance.

The technological innovation in surveillance is another prime indicator of the school-to-prison transformation of schools. For example, facial recognition systems are being rolled out to K–12 and college systems, with large districts like Putnam City School District in Oklahoma having installed the technology in the 2018–19 academic year (Ropek 2019). While these systems are installed to reportedly identify individuals who are not authorized to be on school grounds or identify students in emotional distress for intervention by digitizing students' facial expressions, these databases of digital facial prints are often collected without consent from school visitors or students, or disclosures of how to have your biometric information removed from these databases. Concerns have been raised about the use of emotion-detecting artificial intelligence (AI) technologies as a form of predictive policing, whereby students may be engaged by school authorities before any school infraction occurs, and about false positives that seem to identify particular race-gender intersections more frequently (Buolamwini and Gebru 2018). Some technology providers are now making AI and machine learning–based facial recognition systems available to K–12 districts for free, in hopes of making facial recognition systems a common part of schools' technological infrastructure (Ascione 2019).

It is important to understand the power technology has in shaping social narratives of crime and deviance. For example, decades ago, Ditton (1979) argued that crime waves could in fact reflect innovations in our ability to detect perceived crime rather than changes in rates of offending, and therefore might more appropriately be called "control waves." Advances in technologies of control, an increased reliance on them, along with a hardening of behavioral standards, may be critical components of a recent control wave that has taken place in our schools. Hence, institutional dynamics—rather than increases in deviance—might explain why the STP pipeline has flourished even as rates of school violence have remained stagnant (Muschert et al. 2014; Johnson 2015).

Punishment

Many may consider punishment an outcome produced by carceral education, but it is also a contributing member of the carceral ecosystem in several ways. First, punishment represents a punitive ideology extending from social control. Unlike discipline, punishment sanctions behavior without the steps necessary to secure the internalization of the moral objectives, oftentimes labeling students as "no good" and "troublemakers" instead of reaffirming their potential and the behavioral and attitudinal modifications they need to take to achieve that potential. Without attending to the internalization of codes of moral and character development, punishment may instead increase students' feelings of unfairness, resentment, and the likelihood of future norm violations. Discipline, in contrast, is a process in which school personnel facilitate students' internalization of the moral objectives associated with social sanctions, possibly through modeling due process, and fair and consistent consequences, so that self-regulation will prevent future behavioral violations (R. Bailey et al. 2019).

Second, punishment reflects the excessive and inflexible use of typical disciplinary strategies, including exclusionary discipline (i.e., in-school and out-of-school suspension, expulsion, referrals), humiliation, and corporal punishment (which is still legal in at least nineteen states) to create a strict or harsh school climate. For example, the Race, Gender, and Social Control in STEM Lab found that attending a school that ranked among the top third in its reliance on in-school suspension was related to lowered math scores and rates of college entry for all students, even after controlling for the impact of individual suspensions, school levels of social disorder, and selection into schools (Jabbari and Johnson 2020). Rather than just an outcome, school suspension rates as indicators of climate become potential stressors and determinants of health outcomes.

Third, punishment often includes hegemonic labeling processes that enable a self-fulfilling prophecy to take place. Hegemonic refers to the process through which marginalized populations consciously or unwittingly collude in their own subjugation (Gramsci 1999). According to Howard Becker (1963), "deviance is not the quality of the act the person commits, but rather a consequence of the application by others of rules and sanctions to an offender" (p. 2). Illustrating this point, Ray Rist (1970) explained how a teacher's evaluation of student attributes resulted in students being assigned behavioral labels such as "bright" and "troublemaker." As this process of institutional labeling and student negotiation is repeated over time, Rist argues that student resistance to labeling wanes. The outcome for students is behavioral conformance with the labels of expectation, and for educators the realization of a self-fulfilling prophecy. These processes resemble those documented by Ann Arnett Ferguson (2001) in her analysis of Black boys within STP pipelines. In it, Ferguson highlights processes of "secondary deviation" (to use Rist's language), whereby social reaction or feedback about perceived misconduct led youths to create nondominant status structures in which misconduct became a celebrated identity-marker and strengthened by achieving more serious deviance labels and punishments.

Fourth, dramatic racial disparities in punishment feed racialized narratives about the temperament, nature, and educability of minoritized youths and subsequently beliefs that they are a health threat and undeserving rather than youths who need equitable access to care. Office for Civil Rights (2021) data show minoritized youths face greater penalties for perceived misbehavior in all dimensions of discipline collected in 2017–18. For example, racial disparities in out-of-school and in-school suspensions and transfers to alternative schools show Black students represent between 28 and 38.8 percent of students in each disciplinary category (Office for Civil Rights 2021). Inequitable punishment such as this reifies structural racism by supporting narratives of racial and cultural deficiency and normalizes the experience of punishment-related racial trauma for these communities.

Law Enforcement

The blending of education and the carceral state is facilitated by law enforcement, the courts, and correctional services, but it may be best represented in the presence of school resource officers (SROs), that is, law enforcement and contracted security during school hours. Since the Columbine school shooting in 1999, the funding of officers to remain on school premises during school hours has been a frequent policy response to enhance the safety of schools (Muschert et al. 2014). Data from the National Center for Education Statistics (NCES) found 57 percent of schools had school resource officers on school grounds in the 2015–16 academic year, up from 42 percent just a decade earlier. That number is roughly 70 percent for US high schools (Musu et al. 2019). Additionally, since 2017, K–12 school systems in at least four states (i.e., Texas, Florida, Georgia, Alaska) have added their own police departments. While steps should be taken to prevent horrifying school shootings, police officers on school premises are merely a treatment rather than a solution. In fact, like Sheldon Greenberg's assertion in chapter 7, there is no research showing that the rate of school shootings has declined as the percentage of schools with SROs has increased (Johnson et al. 2019).

Yet the question educational leaders and policymakers should seek answers to regarding SROs is, what are they doing in schools the 99.9 percent of the time they are not intervening with an active shooter? It has been suggested that they are criminalizing typical age-appropriate behavior of children and adolescents while strengthening the STP pipeline (Fasching-Varner et al. 2014). On this point, data show schools with SROs have on average a 12.3 percent higher referral rate than schools without them, and that between 2015 and 2018 school-related arrests and referrals to law enforcement in US schools increased 5 and 12 percent, respectively (Office for Civil Rights 2021). Black students are especially impacted by arrests and referrals; they constitute 28.7 percent of referrals to law enforcement and 31.6 percent of school arrests despite being just 15.1 percent of total school enrollment (Office for Civil Rights 2021). These disparities suggest SROs are contributing to both the school-to-prison transformation and its acute public health implications for Black students.

Neighborhoods: Concentration and Heterogeneity Effects

The disparate impact of carceral education on minoritized students is enabled by the unequal geography of punishment that concentrates social control devices within racially segregated cities and neighborhoods. The geographic concentration of punishment began as Black populations in racially segregated areas saw a heavier police presence after 1970. The exclusion of Blacks from employment in industries and full participation in the housing market effectively confined a large segment of the Black population to relatively few affordable areas where they could be targeted with racist technologies of social control in higher numbers, with greater racial efficiency, and precision (Johnson and Jabbari 2022). Their neighborhoods were subsequently cast—in social science research and political discourse—as socially disorganized and places where drug markets and an associated "underclass" criminality flourished (Grogger and Willis 2000; W. J. Wilson 1997). These narratives laid the foundation for "tough on crime" political decisions that enacted stiffer penalties and zero-tolerance laws to reign in seemingly out-of-control disadvantaged areas (Alexander 2010).

The concentration of disadvantage and punitive state technologies in the racially segregated areas Black families inhabited allowed carceral education to take root in several ways. First, concentrated disadvantage also concentrated kids with the greatest health needs in educational institutions with the greatest tendency to punish those needs. Housing instability (K. M. Ferguson et al. 2012), food insecurity (Kleinman et al. 1998), among other poverty-related conditions became social determinants of both limited opportunities to learn and higher chances of being identified for punishment. Second, the concentration of educational disadvantage that accompanied neighborhood poverty left democratic schools vulnerable to school closure (Ewing 2020), and the opening of charter schools aligned with the no-excuses approach (Burdick-Will et al. 2013). According to 2016 data, 57 percent of charter schools and an overwhelming majority of "no excuses" charter schools are located within urbanized areas (NCES 2018a). The concentration of charter schools in urban areas contributes to city levels of suspension and expulsion at higher rates than traditional public schools (Joseph and CityLab 2016). Third, racial segregation and concentrated poverty are associated with a heavier police presence (Johnson et al. 2019), which contributes to higher neighborhood incarceration rates (Clear 2007) and youth interaction with law enforcement (Shedd 2015). Finally, on this dimension, the School Survey on Crime and Safety reveals recent growth in schools' surveillance methods was greatest in city schools. The use of metal detectors was significantly more likely to be used in city schools than in other locations, even adjusting for neighborhood crime, school size, and the number of violent incidents in school (Addington 2014).

Neighborhoods and schools that are racially and economically heterogeneous are not exempt from carceral education, and in fact they may be used in diverse areas as a means of defending inequities and privilege in access to educational resources. Stratification scholars have long observed that schools with higher White enrollments were among the most stratified because higher-resourced White families demanded it (Jencks and Mayer 1990; Lofton 2021) and were skillful at hoarding resources and opportunities (Lewis-McCoy 2014). Public schools hoping to keep their neighboring White middle-class students from leaving their schools for private options position White students and diversity as beneficiaries of disproportionately high Black suspension and expulsion rates. The empirical work of Johnson and Jabbari (2021) also suggests the consequences of being suspended are greater for Black students in White schools than in Black schools, showing that as the percentage of White enrollment in schools increases, the math scores of Black suspended students decrease until they are significantly lower than the math scores of Black non-suspended students. Therefore, heterogeneous schools may pose a significant risk to the well-being of Black students.

Conclusion

This chapter provided a framework for understanding how social control gives rise to carceral education and its ecosystem, and within them structures such as the STP pipeline that, in turn, pose barriers to the health and well-being of youths, especially those from minoritized communities. This framework has implications for the work of researchers, activists, policymakers, and practitioners, since many of the structures and systems summarized in this review will require action on the part of all parties to replace an ecosystem of risk with one of care and well-being.

What changes are required to secure an ecosystem of care? Answers to this question are implied in the review of each ecosystem domain and are worth summarizing:

- No-excuses charter schools should rethink their commitment to regimented pedagogical practices and strict discipline, as some charter school networks have already announced they would (Golann 2021). Research is needed to understand the experiences of students who were pushed out of no-excuses charters and the average impact that experience had on their physical health and psycho-social well-being.

- Researchers and school systems should evaluate how SROs impact students' mental and physical health, including data on pedestrian police stops that have gone largely unreported in most states. Law enforcement should take on reforms of its own in relation to carceral education as has been done in Philadelphia with some success in reducing student arrests in the 2014–15 school year by 54 percent from a year earlier, and by an additional 64 percent by the next year (Goldstein et al. 2019).

- Policymakers, parents, and activists have a duty to engage schools that mistakenly believe punishment can achieve prosocial youth behavior. Moratoriums on exclusionary discipline have been implemented in large school systems throughout the nation (see Denver, New York, and Los Angeles) to provide schools the opportunity to try other approaches that rely on trauma-informed practices, rehabilitating relationships, and school community inclusion and cohesion.
- State legislatures, state departments of education, and local governments can use Maryland as an example of how to initiate a review of statutes to inform data about youth referrals and racial disproportionalities that arise at each stage of the procedural justice continuum (Young et al. 2011; Governor's Office of Crime Control and Prevention 2019). Legislation should be adopted to curb the penalties of zero-tolerance policy and disturbance laws.
- School systems should delay the adoption of AI technologies in school until processes and innovations are in place that allow individuals to self-select out of digital facial print collection and the probabilities for false positives in identification are equalized across racial groups.
- School systems should review dress code policies to identify and eliminate unnecessary linkages between cultural aesthetics and sanctions and prepare school staff to identify their own biases through anti-racist, anti-bias training.
- It is vitally important that policymakers provide schools serving urban disadvantaged communities with equitable resources and training about how to respond adequately to the health needs of

their students, and trauma-informed educational practices. Expanded access to care in school should coincide with urban renewal in distressed neighborhoods to address community and family stressors that serve as social determinants of learning and student well-being.

By beginning with these points of possible reform, the school-to-prison conversion that is currently underway may be reversed and the health and well-being of all youths, especially minoritized students, can be better supported toward an ecosystem of care and well-being.

7

The Role of School Resource Officers

SHELDON GREENBERG, PHD

School resource officers (SROs) are an increasingly common part of the K–12 public school culture in the United States. School shootings and increased concern about school violence led to growth in SRO programs, with some states requiring schools to employ SROs. The growth in the number of SROs and the proportion of schools and districts employing them has been driven by state policy and federal spending. Since 1998, federal funding to support SROs has exceeded $1 billion. Approximately $14 billion spent to support community policing provided additional funding for SROs (Connery 2020), and the percentage of schools with armed officers grew from 1 percent in 1975 to 58 percent in 2018 (Diliberti et al. 2019).

The use of school resource officers is extremely controversial. Advocates—many of whom are parents of school-age children—cite school violence, mass casualty events, and threats as reason to employ armed officers in schools, including elementary schools. Critics cite the likelihood that vulnerable youth will experience the kind of trauma from interactions with SROs that Odis Johnson cites in chapter 6 and the school-to-prison (STP) pipeline as reasons that schools should not employ armed officers. Nationwide protests over police officer bias and use of force have intensified the debate (Ghavami et al. 2021).

A cornerstone of the debate is a lack of evidence on SRO effectiveness (Mallett 2020). There is very little evidence that the existence of SROs deters crime or violence in schools. Of course, it is difficult to identify and measure crimes that are not committed, but students are very unlikely to report a planned shooting to SROs; they are more likely to trust other school staff. We do know that SROs rarely intervene to stop school violence or school shootings, the primary reason many advocates cite for their existence. In fact, school violence is higher in schools with SROs than schools without SROs (Kupchik 2020; Mowen 2020).

The US Department of Justice (DOJ) and National Association of School Resource Officers (NASRO) define an SRO as "a career law enforcement officer, with sworn authority, deployed in community-oriented policing, and assigned by the employing police department or agency to work in collaboration with schools and community-based organizations" (2022). SROs are defined differently across states and jurisdictions, with statutes in twenty-six states (Connery 2020; Canady 2018). The majority of SROs in the United States are local police officers, deputies, and troopers. Some police officers in schools are members of a school system or district's in-house police department. Some school systems are supporting new or expanded in-house police operations as local police departments relinquish involvement in SRO programs. Other school systems and districts are reducing or eliminating their in-house police agencies (Chen 2022).

The growth in the number of SROs and the different definitions by district or state leads to uncertainty about the number of SROs. Reporting on the number of SROs, including how many schools they serve, how they function, and measures of SRO effectiveness, is not mandated. Based on several studies and self-reporting, the number of SROs is estimated at 46,000, with 58 percent of schools reporting having at least one police officer on site weekly (Diliberti et al. 2019). Twenty-two percent of schools reported having a full-time SRO, and 21 percent reported the presence of a part-time SRO. Approximately 68 percent of high schools, 59 percent of middle schools, and 30 percent of elementary schools reported having an SRO present at least once each week (National Association of Secondary School Principals 2020). NASRO estimates the number of SROs to be smaller, closer to 20,000, based on enrollment in basic SRO training (NASRO 2020b).

SROs are not distributed randomly. They are disproportionately placed in schools that are predominantly Black or Hispanic. High schools with a population composed of 25 to 50 percent Black and/or Hispanic students had a higher rate of SROs than schools with 10 percent or fewer Black or Hispanic students (Lindsay et al. 2018). This fact only increases the concern of those who cite the negative impact of the school-to-prison pipeline in these districts and the disproportionate impact on vulnerable populations. Additionally, because SROs are not required to be trained in asset-based approaches or be experts in mental health education, the fact that they are more likely to encounter underrepresented minority (URM) students is of great concern to public health and educational experts. As a result, there is a call for action, led by organizations such as Police Free Schools and the American Civil Liberties Union, to remove all police officers from schools to reduce the STP pipeline, overresponse to discipline, and infringement on student rights.

Brief History

The assignment of police officers to schools began in the 1950s in Flint, Michigan. The initial effort was called the Police-School Liaison Program (S. Wilson 2016). The Flint program became a national model, but the concept of assigning officers to schools was a slow process. In 1973, the Justice Department's National Advisory Commission on Criminal Justice Standards and Goals recommended that police agencies promote the concept of placing officers in schools. The commission recommended that law enforcement agencies with over four hundred employees assign a full-time officer to every junior and senior high school to teach, counsel, be a resource to school officials, and enforce law (National Legal Aid and Defender Association 1973).

Also, in the 1970s, several large school systems obtained legislation to establish their own police departments. Staffed by sworn/certified police officers, also called SROs, these departments operated under the control of the school system or district, independent of local or state law enforcement agencies. The largest of the school police agencies was the Los Angeles County School District Police Department. Other school system police departments were established in Baltimore (MD), Dade County (FL), Philadelphia (PA), San Bernardino (CA), Clark County (NV), and other jurisdictions. Some large police and sheriff's departments, particularly those in urban areas, began assigning officers to schools primarily to teach about substance abuse, avoiding gangs, and traffic safety.

In the early 1990s, the Department of Justice through the Improving America's Schools Act provided funding to police departments to support SROs (Lindberg 2015). In 1991, NASRO was formed and adopted a triad approach, focusing on the role of SROs as teacher, counselor, and law enforcement officer. Demands to establish SRO presence and other security measures expanded throughout the 1990s after the shooting at Columbine High School and other mass casualty events (Weiler and Cray 2011).

While active shooter events and fear of mass shootings played a role in the expansion of SRO programs, mass casualty events in schools remain rare (Federal Bureau of Investigation 2020). Data on active shooter events in schools compiled by the Center for Homeland Defense and Security at the Naval Postgraduate School shows that SROs played a role in many of the crises. SROs were on duty in 49 percent of the school attacks, responding within one minute in 29 percent of the situations. Moreover, SROs ended the attack in 12 percent of the situations. The presence of an SRO decreased the duration of active shooter incidents from eight to two minutes (Reidman and O'Neill 2019).

Historically, police service to schools that do not have SROs has been provided by beat or area patrol officers. As noted above, there is little evidence of the role patrol officers play in supporting prevention and intervention efforts in schools. Except for training on active shooter situations, there is no data or research on uniformed patrol officer preparedness or readiness to engage with schools (Greenberg 2017).

Role of SROs and Variation in SRO Programs

There is significant variety in the role SROs play in schools and districts. There is support for placing a trained officer in every school as a "layer of security for prevention and response in the case of an active threat on a school campus" (Hutchinson 2013; NASRO 2020a). Some states (e.g., Florida, Maryland, and South Carolina) have called for SROs (or security officers) to be assigned to every school, although there is no evidence to support that all schools need or would benefit from their presence (Raymond 2010). The merit of assigning police officers to every school continues to be debated (Corley 2018). There is also a wide variance in how SROs function. Their role varies based in part on the school culture and school administrators who interact with the officers (McKenna et al. 2016). School administrators expect that SROs in their schools will provide expanded safety, improved perceptions of safety, and reduce interruptions for teachers (Raymond 2010). School and police administrators often establish SRO programs based on memoranda of understanding (MOUs) or memoranda of agreement (MOAs). These agreements establish the parameters for the position, citing duties and restrictions. An SRO program may, however, be established without formal agreement, policy, or guidelines (Counts et al. 2018).

But most SROs are full-time police officers who are trained to meet the same performance requirements of other officers in their department. In some schools, the role of SRO is filled by retired officers and private security personnel who do not have to meet standards established by the local police department. In both cases, their training may not extend to topics such as mental health, adolescent development, or education curriculum. Because SRO duties to schools are in addition to their core function as law enforcement officers (Rosiak 2009) and SROs are often evaluated according to the same criteria as cops who walk a beat, you can understand that they may not deliver the outcomes that school or district leaders expect.

Beyond their training, the fact that SROs work for their law enforcement agency also affects their abilities. They do not work for school principals or school systems (Price 2008). They may be assigned by their agency to one or more schools. A large high school may have one or more SROs assigned on a full-time basis. Within the same jurisdiction, one SRO may have responsibility for three or more schools. Regardless of the number of schools to which they are assigned, SROs may assume roles as a teacher, counselor, enforcer of laws and rules, security officer, and an "extra pair of hands" for school administrators (Thurau and Wald 2009; Bernardy and

Schmid 2018). Measuring the many tasks SROs perform beyond crime prevention, crime intervention, teaching, and counseling is difficult (McKenna and Pollock 2014). Policies and procedures that define how SROs should intervene in matters related to student misbehavior are lacking (Ryan et al. 2018). SROs are first responders to calls from teachers, administrators, staff, and students. They respond to routine or nonserious student behavioral and disciplinary matters. While 79 percent of SROs report not being involved in school discipline, research shows that the majority involve themselves based on their knowledge of teachers and staff, of the circumstance, and the involved students (Curran et al. 2019). A challenging piece of the SRO puzzle is the number and complexity of tasks that SROs are asked to perform in schools, sometimes without much training. These range from patrolling the hallways and cafeterias, to responding to crises and serious incidents, to providing emergency management training.

Qualifications and Selection of SROs

Placing an SRO in a school requires planning, a structured selection process, specialized and ongoing training, policies and procedures, effective communication, and a system for assessing performance. It requires placement of officers who can adapt to the school culture and work well with students, teachers, counselors, administrators, parents, and others (S. Clark 2011). Selection of SROs is determined primarily by the officer's law enforcement agency. Data on the criteria used by agencies to identify and select SROs are lacking. Generally, principals and other school officials play little or no role in the selection process. As a result, the officer's "fit" into the school environment may take time to evolve. Timely and smooth transition and integration; development of positive relations with students, teachers, counselors, nurses, and others; and successful performance are achieved more efficiently when school officials play a role in the SRO selection process (Canady 2018).

Training, Preparedness, and Readiness

The extent to which SROs are trained and oriented to the culture of the schools varies. Training is required in some jurisdictions but is merely recommended in others. NASRO recommends that training occurs before SROs are assigned to schools, however some police agencies and school systems allow officers to be assigned prior to training. In states in which there is no legislation or policy requiring instruction, officers may be placed in schools with no SRO-related training throughout their tenure. Data on the number of SROs who received training specific to the role are lacking.

The most recognized training for SROs is the NASRO Basic Course and NASRO twenty-four-hour advanced course. Among the topics in which additional SRO training is needed are managing student behavior, engaging in nonserious disciplinary matters, managing fear, de-escalation, intervening in mental health crises, enforcing zero-tolerance policies, interacting with students of color and those who have disabilities, and preventing gang recruitment (Merkwae 2015). SRO training is required in twenty-eight states and the District of Columbia. The District of Columbia and fifteen states require both training and certification. Maryland, Utah, and Virginia are the only states known to mandate SRO training on implicit bias and diversity awareness (Z. Perez and Erwin 2020). Virginia, Massachusetts, Washington, New York, and California are among states that legislated standards and training for SROs. Required training in Virginia, for example, addresses working with youths, school safety, school law, and SRO responsibilities. The state's mandated courses include crisis management, adolescent brain development, working with special needs populations, implicit bias, mediation, and the effect of trauma (Virginia Department of Criminal Justice Services 2021). The State of Texas passed legislation in 2015 requiring school districts with at least 30,000 students to train SROs on de-escalation, mental and behavioral health, crisis intervention, child and adolescent development, conflict resolution, and restorative justice (S. Wilson 2016).

SRO Effectiveness

Despite growth in SRO programs over the past twenty years, little is known about the effectiveness of SROs in preventing crime and disorder and increasing safety in schools (Kenneth Anderson 2018). There is limited research on the impact of SROs on student discipline and academic outcomes

(Weisburst 2019). Despite the lack of evidence, there is general support for and belief in the effectiveness of SROs from school principals and police executives (Chrusciel et al. 2015; T. Gregory 2018; Finn and McDevitt 2005). Perspectives vary on SROs and reduction of school violence. There is limited research on whether SROs reduce or exacerbate fear of harm. Critics of SRO programs suggest that their presence leads to increased exclusionary discipline, such as suspension, expulsion, and arrest (Fisher and Hennessy 2016).

There is a dearth of research on SRO success, the number and type of incidents they prevent, and how they intervene (Raymond 2010; Weiler and Cray 2011; Daniels et al. 2011; Agnich 2015). It is difficult to measure the crimes and other high-risk situations that SROs prevent (Esserman 2018). Additionally, there is limited evidence showing that SROs deter school shootings (D. Goldstein 2020; James and McCallion 2013). The National Averted School Violence Database, operated by the National Police Foundation, has only gathered limited data. An averted school violence incident is defined as a violent attack planned with or without the use of a firearm that was prevented either before or after the potential perpetrator arrived at school grounds and before any injury or loss of life occurred. Information reported to the database is provided on a voluntary basis. Of the incidents in the database, 58.8 percent were prevented by a police officer who intervened or received information from a student or other source about a pending violent act (Daniels 2019).

Evidence on SRO effectiveness in preventing bullying also is limited (Devlin et al. 2018). SRO intervention in bullying incidents may be classified in reports as threat, harassment, or assault. SROs are not required to report on informal interactions with those who commit or are victimized by bullying. Limited evidence can also be attributed to a lack of common or accepted definitions of school-based incidents, the small number of serious situations that occur in schools, and lack of mandated, centralized, and consistent reporting. Much of the information on SRO effectiveness is anecdotal, thus there is a need for increased research on SRO performance (Weiler and Cray 2011).

SROs and the School-to-Prison Pipeline

As noted in other chapters in this book, the school-to-prison pipeline is a phenomenon in which students become involved in the criminal justice system as a result of policies and practices that use law enforcement rather than traditional school discipline to address behavioral problems (Owens 2017). The presence of police officers in schools has led to disproportionately higher suspension, expulsion, and arrest of Black, Hispanic, and Native American students, and students who have special needs (Lindsay et al. 2018; Gottfredson et al. 2020; D. Goldstein 2020; Mallett 2017). The school-to-prison pipeline has short- and long-term negative impact on students, especially those from marginalized populations and those who have special needs (Nance 2016). A critical issue is that students may engage in crime and disorder during the time they are away from school (Cuellar and Markowitz 2015). Removing students from school due to suspension or expulsion doubles the probability of them becoming involved in situations that result in arrest (Curran 2016).

The role of SROs has evolved from reducing violence and preventing mass casualty events to include tasks such as teaching, counseling, and intervening in classroom management issues (D. Goldstein 2020). In some schools, particularly those in which teachers and staff are in fear due to constant or excessive challenge, SROs are called to situations that in most circumstances would not involve police. Whether these roles are consistent with their training and how students perceive them is an important question and answered to some degree by the work of other chapter authors, including Odis Johnson and Richard Lofton. SRO response may elevate student misbehavior to a criminal or delinquent act, propelling students into the justice system (B. Brown 2018). SRO involvement in classroom management and non-criminal disciplinary matters has contributed to excessive discipline and the school-prison-pipeline, particularly involving Black, Hispanic, and Native American male and female students, poor students, and students who have disabilities (Counts et al. 2018; Pentek and Eisenberg 2018).

When called, SROs follow legal and policy mandates, training, and rely on experience and intuition when determining an action, which may include arrest (Wolf 2014). The result of SROs following their training is a larger number of nonserious violent offenses (Na and Gottfredson 2013). A study by the Council of State Governments found that schools with SROs experienced a 12.3 percent increase in nonserious violent crimes reported to police and that SRO presence leads to more arrests for disorderly conduct than arrests for assault and weapon charges (E. Morgan et al. 2014).

SROs are often called upon to enact zero-tolerance policies in schools with large numbers of vulnerable adolescents. Zero tolerance is a philosophical approach to discipline that mandates predetermined consequences—most often suspension or expulsion—for violations of certain rules, regardless of circumstances or situational context (Welch and Payne 2018). Zero-tolerance policies—which are in direct opposition to asset-based approaches like restorative practice, as described in chapters 5 and 6—often compel teachers and school officials to engage police officers in situations that may not warrant law enforcement intervention. The rapid reliance on SROs in zero-tolerance situations contributes to inordinate discipline of students of color and the school-to-prison pipeline (Welsh and Little 2018; Curran 2016). To date, there is little evidence that zero-tolerance policies have achieved intended objectives (Welch and Payne 2018).

Innovative and alternative approaches to extreme discipline have the potential to end the school-to-prison pipeline, strengthen equity, and enhance the learning environment. Alternative approaches, including limiting SRO involvement, rethinking zero tolerance, and restorative justice practices, can reduce criminalizing typical adolescent developmental behaviors and low-level offenses such as acting out in class, engaging in peer conflicts, failing to obey teacher directives, and being truant (Schiff 2018; Mallett 2016).

Future of SRO Programs

Support for SROs is driven by school shootings, increases in other violence, and fear. Political leaders often react to shootings in schools by calling for additional SROs. Laws such as the Stop School Violence Act continue to provide funding for SRO programs and other security measures (US Department of Justice 2021). On the one hand, educational groups such as the National Parent Teacher Association (PTA), the National Association of School Psychologists (NASP), the American School Counselor Association (ASCA), and the National Association of Secondary School Principals (NASSP) support police officers in schools, but they seek change in standards, selection processes, training, and data collection. On the other hand, incidents of excessive force and bias by officers in the community and in schools intensify the call to end SRO programs. Organizations including Police Free Schools, Black Lives Matter, the Healthy Schools Campaign, Alliance for Educational Justice, and the Advancement Project support ending police presence in schools.

Among the controversial issues that exist when reviewing the inclusion of SROs is their role in advancing equity and reducing adverse impact on students based on race, color, ethnicity, and gender; consistent and thorough reporting on SRO activity; mandatory training prior to SRO assignment to schools; and expanded SRO training. The little research on SROs that has been done has had little impact on politics and people's emotions related to school safety. While the debate continues over the value of SROs, federal funding to support their placement remains. As in the past, major incidents such as the mass shooting at Robb Elementary School in Uvalde, Texas, will renew calls for police officers in schools and advance school-based security technologies nationwide, regardless of the evidence.

Conclusion

Predicting the future of police officers in schools is difficult. Placement of SROs will remain a contentious issue based on public perceptions, inconsistencies in the role and across jurisdictions, adverse impacts on students of color and others, the school-to-prison pipeline, and lack of evidence on SRO performance and outcomes (Rosiak 2018). Public sentiment has varied, and momentum to maintain or increase SRO presence has both waned and grown in recent years (Dianis 2021). New and improved evidence on the effectiveness of SRO programs is needed and will guide decision-making on SROs in schools.

8

Restorative Practices

ASHLEY A. GRANT, PHD, OLIVIA MARCUCCI, PHD,
AND DOUGLAS J. MAC IVER, PHD

In an ideal world, schools are supposed to be safe and healthy communities where students can learn and develop. For many children, they serve that function. But for some—often students in urban areas, students from poor families, and students of color—schools overly rely on prison-like procedures, rules, rewards, and punishments to control the movement and behavior of students (Noguera 2003). These punishment-focused schools do not optimize safety, health, or student learning. In recent years, some stakeholders have pushed back against this maximum-security approach to maintaining discipline. Instead, they advocate for a restorative approach to discipline, grounded in restorative justice (RJ), a philosophy that focuses on maintaining resilient communities by repairing harm to relationships when a wrongdoing occurs (Zehr 2015). This chapter reviews the evidence about how RJ and corresponding restorative practices (i.e., how RJ is implemented in schools) contribute to safe, healthy, and socially just schools. After an overview of school discipline and safety in the United States, the chapter summarizes the philosophy and dissemination of RJ and restorative practices (RPs) in schools. Finally, this chapter reviews effectiveness research on RPs, focusing on one of the most recent and comprehensive multicity studies.

A Brief History of Approaches to Safety (and Discipline) in US (Urban) Schools

Traditionally, schools in the United States have relied on punitive practices and policies to create orderly and safe environments. Punitive approaches to safety historically took one of two forms: *corporal* punishment or *exclusionary* punishment. While corporal punishment in schools is still legal in some states, it fell out of favor in the middle of the twentieth century (Kaitlin Anderson 2018). Since the civil rights movement—and particularly since the popularization of zero-tolerance policies in the 1990s—schools now rely on *exclusionary* punishment to create safe learning environments. Federal legislation like the Gun-Free Schools Act of 1994 accelerated a wave of state and local legislation that institutionalized the use of exclusionary discipline in schools (United States Congress 1993; Mongan and Walker 2012). Exclusionary discipline relies on physical and social exclusion in response to a perceived student misbehavior. The most researched exclusionary punishment in schools includes suspensions and expulsions; however, exclusionary discipline also includes sending students to sit in the hallway, to the principal's office, or any disciplinary actions that removes a student from the learning environment. In 2018, 2,529,571 K–12 public school students received an in-school suspension (5% of the public-school population), and 2,419,101 received an out-of-school suspension (4.8% of the school population) (US Department of Education 2021b). As highlighted in chapters 6 and 7, the rise of exclusionary practices is also associated with the use of school resource officers (i.e., a fully qualified police officers assigned to a school community; see Fisher and Hennessy 2016). In 2018, more than 50 percent of schools reported having a school resource officer (Diliberti et al. 2019).

As with the decline of corporal punishment in schools, prominent scholars, activists, community members, and educators are now critiquing exclusionary punishment as both ineffective and harmful (American Psychological Association Zero Tolerance Task Force 2008). While suspensions and other extreme exclusionary policies were originally created to respond to extreme or violent misbehavior, they are now instead more likely to be implemented for minor misbehaviors or disruptions (Vavrus and Cole 2002). This mismatch between (mis)behavior and consequence leads to schools that focus disproportionately on controlling student bodies and behavior rather than student learning or community healing (Noguera 2003). Students who are suspended are more likely to drop out, less likely to be civically engaged as adults, and more likely to be both the perpetrator and victim of a crime, along with other serious, lifelong consequences (Wolf and Kupchik 2017; T. Lee et al. 2011). In addition, there is growing evidence of the collateral damage of suspensions: even students who *are not* disciplined but attend high-suspension schools have lower math achievement, reading achievement, and college attendance (Jabbari and Johnson 2020; Perry and Morris 2014).

Ineffectiveness and harmfulness are serious concerns, yet exclusionary discipline also leads to greater inequity. "Hyper-disciplining" refers to the disproportionate targeting (conscious or unconscious) of students according to race, ethnicity, class, ability status, and more, even when controlling for rates of misbehavior (Marcucci 2020). In their conceptual piece on safety and discipline, Johnson and colleagues (2019) argue that exclusionary disciplinary practices have increased racial disparities in discipline in schools. Other research supports this claim. Compared to their White peers, Black and Indigenous students are hyper-disciplined (Sprague et al. 2013; Skiba, Chung, et al. 2014). Research on Hispanic students is more mixed, given the racial diversity of the population, though many large-scale sophisticated analyses find that Hispanic students are hyper-disciplined up to around 2.5 times their White peers (Cruz and Rodl 2018; Skiba, Horner, et al. 2011). Despite much research showing that Asian American or Pacific Islander students are underrepresented in the disciplinary pipeline (Skiba, Horner, et al. 2011, 85–107; Skiba, Chung, et al. 2014; Cruz and Rodl 2018), when disaggregated from their Asian peers, Pacific Islanders are hyper-disciplined as well (Nguyen et al. 2019). Additionally, male students, students with disabilities, and lesbian, gay, bisexual, trans, and queer students receive harsher sanctions for misbehavior (Mittleman 2018b; Welsh and Little, 2018). Students with multiple intersecting identities in these targeted populations have an even greater risk for exclusion (Annamma et al. 2019). While scholars have been drawing attention to this hyper-disciplining since 1975 (Children's Defense Fund 1975), the federal government officially released a "Dear Colleague" letter in 2014 outlining the civil rights violations of these exclusionary discipline responses and suggesting actions school systems can take to ameliorate them (US Department of Justice and US Department of Education 2014). Given these serious critiques of exclusionary discipline, a new philosophy is beginning to take hold: restorative justice.

Brief Description and History of Restorative Practices in Schools

Restorative justice is a philosophy rooted in diverse Indigenous epistemologies, with specific practices stemming in part from Navajo tribes (North America) and Māori communities (New Zealand) (Sellman et al. 2013; Zehr 2015). As Winn (2018) writes, "restorative justice is not merely an alternative to punishment; it is a way of life . . . [it is] a paradigm shift" (p. 18). The social discipline window (figure 8.1) positions restorative justice along with other approaches to discipline (Wachtel and McCold 2001).

Unlike the punitive paradigm (which includes exclusionary discipline), the restorative philosophy has both high expectations and support for students. Many theoretical traditions, including social control theory and libertarian justice theory, support the idea that a restorative philosophy can create safe and healthy schools (Hirschi 2001; Grant and Mac Iver 2021). Accordingly, this chapter asserts that high-quality relationships and equity are the building blocks for creating safe and healthy schools—and that restorative justice creates space for both relationships and equity

Restorative justice refers to the overarching paradigm, or philosophy; restorative practices (RPs) are how educators put RJ into practice in schools. Specifically, RPs are a collection of habitual approaches and procedures intended to (1) build community by fostering dialogue, understanding, problem solving, and developing equitable relationships; (2) prevent hurtful behavior and conflict such as bullying, violence, and injustice; and (3) effectively repair harm, prevent recurrence of harm, provide just consequences, and restore relationships.

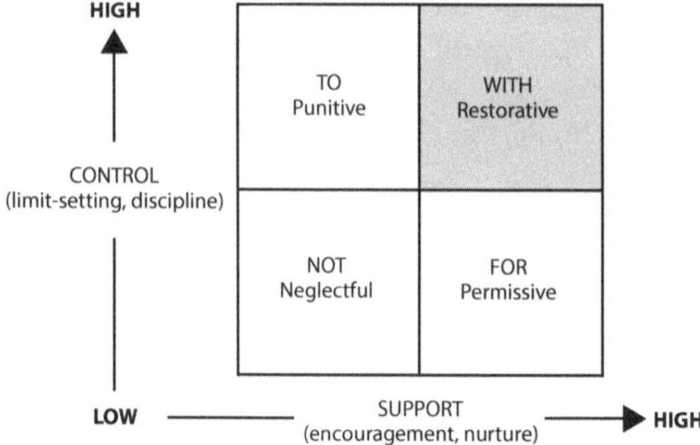

Figure 8.1 Simplified social discipline window.
Source: From Wachtel and McCold 2001, "Restorative Justice in Everyday Life." Copyright © International Institute for Restorative Practices. All rights reserved. Used with permission.

In schools, RPs fall along a spectrum from informal to formal (Wachtel and McCold 2001). Informal RPs include affective statements and restorative questions, where an educator uses a restorative philosophy to guide interactions with students. Formal RPs include circle processes, where a group comes together in a circle to engage in a structured dialogue or conflict resolution (Pranis 2005). Circles can be proactive—aimed at building community—or responsive—aimed at repairing harm. A proactive circle, sometimes referred to as talking or community circles, is implemented regularly within a classroom to strengthen and maintain relationships. A responsive circle—including peace circles, restorative mediation, and reentry circles—is held after a wrongdoing occurs (Pranis 2005). All RPs, regardless of their position on the formal/informal axis or the proactive or responsive axis, are based on dialogue and relationship building.

Dissemination of RP in Schools

The adoption of RPs in schools began in Australia and New Zealand (Karp and Breslin 2001). The first recorded use of a restorative practice in a school context occurred in 1994 in Queensland, Australia, after an assault at a school dance (Cameron and Thorsborne 2001). From there, schools across the world began implementing RPs and restorative philosophies (Reimer 2018; McCluskey et al. 2008). Although some adoptions of RPs have come under criticism for implementing the *practices* without the necessary philosophical shift (Vaandering 2010), the use of RPs continues to grow. Between 2015 and 2017, the number of schools in the United States that reported using restorative circles increased from 30.9 percent to 41.6 percent (M. Jackson et al. 2018; Diliberti et al. 2019). The same nationally representative data found that restorative circles are more common in urban schools, compared to rural and suburban schools (Diliberti et al. 2019). Indeed, most urban centers across the country now include RPs in their approach to school climate.

This spread of RPs within the United States has been supported in large part by the work of the International Institute for Restorative Practices (IIRP). Since the graduate school institution was founded in the 2000s, IIRP has been at the forefront of disseminating RPs to schools and other institutions, training over 10,000 educators (International Institute for Restorative Practices 2020). Specifically, IIRP has created a whole-school model of RPs called SaferSanerSchools, which focuses on school climate improvement. The next section addresses some of the critiques of the SaferSanerSchools model, as well as research on effectiveness of RPs overall.

Effectiveness of RPs in Schools

Some critics misinterpret RPs in general—and SaferSanerSchools specifically—as over-permissive approaches that lead to disorder. However, RPs have been shown to reduce discipline severity and the use of suspensions, as well as to improve school climate and teacher and student attendance (Darling-Hammond et al. 2020; Weber and Vereenooghe 2020). Currently, most of the evidence about the outcomes of school-based RPs relies on observational research designs and, thus, less reliable evidence. Although these studies cannot be used to make causal statements, they still provide compelling evidence that RPs can positively impact schools. For example, Anyon and colleagues' (2016) study of the well-established RPs in Denver Public Schools found that exposure to a restorative practice in the first semester of the school year was associated with a reduced risk of suspension later in the year. In their qualitative case study of an urban high school, González et al. (2019) found that student leadership in restorative initiatives can democratize schools. Other observational studies have generated evidence that school-based RPs can mitigate the hyper-disciplining of marginalized students (González 2015), reduce absenteeism (Armour 2012), and improve school climate and safety (A. Gregory et al. 2016), among other outcomes. Importantly, some district-specific analyses have shown an association between RPs and increased academic outcomes, including math and reading standardized test scores (Armour 2012; Kerstetter 2016). In an evaluation of Oakland Unified School District's RPs, Jain et al. (2014) even found that graduation rates increased in restorative schools compared to non-restorative schools. This type of research has led to a promising body of evidence that supports the positive impacts of school-based restorative justice.

Importantly, a few randomized, controlled trials have supplemented the developing research based on school-based RPs. The SaferSanerSchools model from IIRP, introduced in the previous section, was evaluated in a randomized, controlled trial in Pittsburgh Public Schools (PPS) (Augustine et al. 2018). Forty-four schools in PPS were randomly assigned to implement the SaferSanerSchools model. After two years, teachers in the restorative schools reported a better school climate compared to teachers in the control schools. In addition, restorative schools reduced their overall rates of suspension and reduced the hyper-disciplining of Black students and of low-income students. While many of the results indicated a positive influence of the whole-school restorative model, the study did find some areas that were not affected, such as suspension rates among male students or students with disabilities. On top of that, some negative effects were documented in the middle grades, which saw no changes to suspension rates and worse academic outcomes (Augustine et al. 2018). Although the impact of RP on students' mental well-being or social-emotional growth remains an area that needs more investigation, another randomized control trial found schools using RPs reduced bullying, which makes sense given their focus on improving relationships (Bonnell et al. 2018).

The Augustine et al. study, along with a few other isolated, randomized, controlled trials (Acosta et al. 2019; Bonnell et al. 2018) and the observational studies described above, provide preliminary research that a restorative justice paradigm can create safe and healthy schools. One cautionary theme that comes through in all the studies (including the one discussed below), is the large investment in time and effort required by schools implementing RPs. Without this investment, the shift in thinking about disciplinary response required by RP is not always actualized (Lustick 2017) and without the proper supports RP can feel like a burden and not provide true justice for victims (Alvis 2015). The remainder of the chapter focuses on reviewing results from a major, multicity randomized controlled trial that comments on this and attends to some of these gaps in the literature.

Current Study: Restorative Practices with Diplomas Now in Eight US Cities

To this evidence, this chapter adds evidence from the study by the team at Johns Hopkins University that examined the impacts of the SaferSanerSchools RP model when it was integrated with Diplomas Now, a whole-school reform model. The RP substudy involved thirty-three low-performing middle and high schools in eight of the largest urban US districts, representing multiple US regions (New England, Mid-Atlantic, South, Southeast, Midwest, and West). The schools in the sample predominantly enrolled students from traditionally underserved backgrounds: 96 percent of students were from minoritized racial groups and 77 percent from low-income backgrounds.

The SaferSanerSchools Model within a Diplomas Now Framework

Beginning in 2010–11, sixty-two middle and high schools in eleven districts began participating in a randomized controlled trial (experiment) of the whole-school turnaround model Diplomas Now (DN; see Corrin et al. 2014 for full details on DN). In 2014, eight districts agreed to enhance and extend the original study to test the impacts of a more comprehensive model ("RP w/DN") that integrated IIRP's SaferSanerSchools model into the schools previously randomly assigned to DN. Control schools remained in the "other reforms/business as usual" condition. In the RP w/DN schools, the full-time, on-site "transformation facilitator" overseeing DN's support systems became the key person supporting RP implementation. Trainers and coaches from IIRP assisted these facilitators in implementing RP by providing whole-school training sessions, handbooks and other resources, follow-up site visits and telephone consultations, and the formation of professional learning groups of teachers and staff focused on mastering and implementing the eleven essential elements of RP (figure 8.2).

Impacts of RP with DN

This study tested how RP w/DN created a more safe and healthy school as indicated by reductions in suspensions, problematic behavior, violence, and absenteeism, and school climate improvements. It specifically tackles the policy-relevant question: what happens when schools are assigned to implement RP, regardless of how well individual schools do so? The study found that there was

1. **Less exclusionary discipline**—The RP w/DN intervention significantly reduced the probability that students would be suspended three or more days ($p < .05$). Specifically, students at RP w/DN schools were 34 percent less likely than students at control schools to be suspended these many days. We focused on the outcome of "three or more days suspended," because it better captures how successful a school is at preventing major and persistent episodes of problem behavior. For example, it indicates that students did not commit major violations (resulting in more than two days of exclusion) or become persistent violators (earning multiple minor exclusions, totaling three days or more). Contrary to some of the popular rhetoric around the elimination of consequences that can accompany RP, our findings indicated that in RP w/DN schools, a brief one-time exclusion was sometimes viewed as a just and helpful consequence. For example, a one-day exclusion was used as a "cooling off and reflection day" while the school planned and

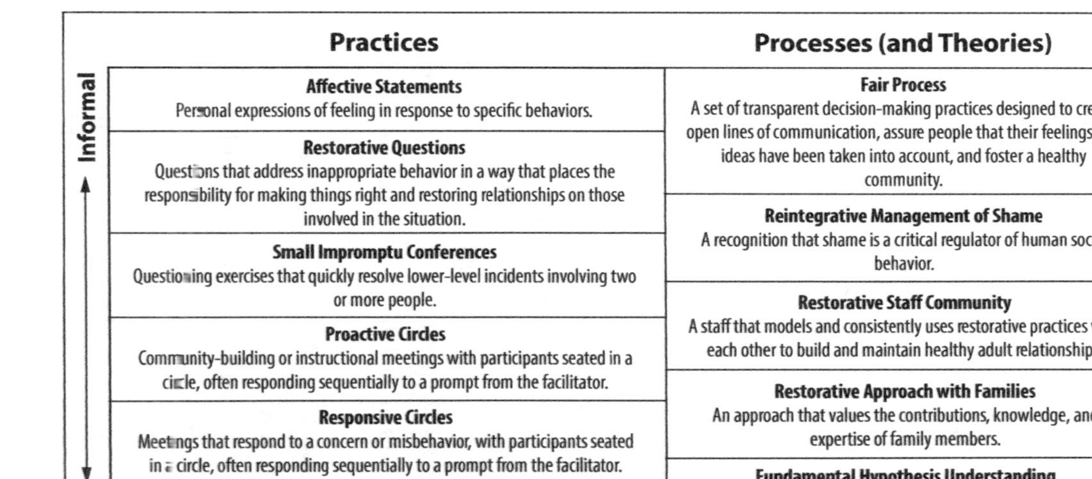

Figure 8.2 11 essential elements of RP

Source: Copyright © International Institute for Restorative Practices. All rights reserved. Used with permission.

arranged a restorative conference to bring affected parties together for discussion of the harms that occurred and to mutually agree on further actions to make things right and mend damaged relationships.

2. **Fewer problematic behaviors and less violence**—Students in RP w/DN schools reported feeling safer, as captured by their reports of how big of a problem troubling behaviors and violence were in their schools. Students were specifically asked about ten types of incidents, including teacher victimization, verbal abuse, fights, vandalism, and thefts. On average, students in control schools reported that these issues were about halfway between "a small problem" and "a medium problem." In RP w/DN schools, students reported these issues were closer to being a small problem (impact estimate, $b = -0.12$, $p = .02$; effect size, $ES = -0.13$).
3. **Less chronic absenteeism**—The study examined chronic absenteeism—when a student has a school attendance rate below 90 percent—to understand how RP impacted students' engagement in school, a key element of a healthy school experience. Students in RP w/DN schools were 20 percent less likely to become chronic absentees than students in control schools, although this impact was only marginally significant statistically ($p < .10$). This provides some evidence to support our original hypothesis that a shift from a punitive approach to a restorative, community-building approach could improve engagement and attendance, by enhancing relationships, school climate, and a sense of being a valued member of the school community whose voice was important. Long-term, improved student attendance benefits students individually (with improved grades and greater chances of graduation) and benefits the school (facilitating community building and learning).
4. **More positive school climate**—Finally, the study analyzed how the RP w/DN intervention impacted teachers' and students' feelings about the school environment, particularly looking at their ratings of school climate, overall and on specific subdomains. Overall, teachers in schools assigned to RP w/DN reported more

> positive perceptions of school climate ($p < .10$, $ES = 0.27$) than teachers in control schools, driven by how it enhanced teachers' sense of professional learning and collaboration ($p < .05$, $ES = 0.20$). Similarly, students in the intervention schools reported more positive overall perceptions of school climate ($p < .05$, $ES = 0.15$), due largely to how the intervention created a more supportive social environment ($p < .10$, $ES = .15$) and reduced problematic behaviors ($p < .05$, $ES = .12$).

See Grant 2020; Grant et al. 2023; and Grant, Mac Iver, and Mac Iver 2022, for more technical details on the study's analyses and findings.

Lessons for Practice: Variability and Implementation

Like with many policies or experiments, implementation of the RP assignment varied among the schools in our study—schools assigned to RP did not use all of the training or supports as designed, nor did they all utilize RP practices at the same high levels. For example, of the seventeen RP schools in our study, two chose to receive local RP support (from their district's Restorative Justice office) rather than support from IIRP and three received supports in the first year but declined continued services from IIRP after the start of the second (2015–16) school year (in order to focus on other professional development [PD] topics). Among the remaining twelve schools who received IIRP support through the full two years of the study, half received all four PD training days. Looking at the usage of RP, teachers and students in schools assigned to RP used and observed others using it more than teachers and students in control schools ($ES = .18$ and $.13$, respectively). Interestingly though, RP practices and professional development were common among many schools not assigned to RP; for example, almost half of the teachers in the control group reported receiving three kinds of PD related to RP and two-thirds of teachers in the larger sample reported at least sometimes using circles to respond to problems. This suggests that impacts of RP may be underestimated in this study due to control group teachers who had been exposed to RP previously and employed some RP-like approaches.

The variability in actual RP usage is reflected in the impact estimates. Although most of the *average* treatment effects were statistically significant in the positive direction, individual schools and blocks varied widely in how much they used RP and in the impact of RP assignment on the outcomes described above. This variability is important for administrators and policymakers to incorporate into their planning of RP implementation and reinforces the necessity of needs and readiness assessments during these early stages (Garnett et al. 2020).

Although we cannot draw causal inferences about the impact of these variations in implementation on schools' outcomes (since schools were not randomly assigned to varied levels of RP), we have conducted exploratory follow-up analyses to better understand this relationship and to help provide suggestive evidence for practitioners and policymakers. In these analyses, we observed a link between more frequent RP implementation and more positive school climate. In particular, the amount of RP-related PD that teachers reported receiving consistently linked with both more positive school climate and their greater intentions to remain teaching at their school. Additionally, looking at the sample from this study as a whole—regardless of a school's status as a treatment or control school—teachers who used more RP themselves were also more likely to intend to stay at their school. (See Grant, 2020, for more details on these studies.)

Conclusion

This chapter summarizes the evidence about the effectiveness of RP to create a safe and healthy school environment. Recent experimental evidence supports many of the encouraging earlier findings from less rigorous studies that show that RPs in schools promote a more positive school climate and reduce the reliance on exclusionary discipline. This chapter particularly discussed findings from the study of RP w/DN, which adds important new evidence about the effectiveness of RP to reduce suspensions, chronic absenteeism, and problematic behaviors and to improve school climate. The study adds to our knowledge about RP due to its randomized design (for stronger claims about cause and effect), sampling across eight different US cities (for potential greater generalizability), and implementation among schools with high need of turnaround (for greater policy relevance). The promise of RP is strong to help create safe and healthy learning environments in US urban schools, but more research is needed, particularly studies that focus on enhancing and sustaining implementation and long-term effects of RP.

9

K–12 Schools in the United States during the COVID-19 Pandemic: Public Health Mitigation, Equity Considerations, and the Impact of Education Disruption on the Nation's Most Disadvantaged Youths

MEGAN COLLINS, MD, MPH, SARA JOHNSON, PHD, MPH, ALAN REGENBERG, MBE, ANNETTE ANDERSON, PHD, MS, BETH MARSHALL, DRPH, MPH, ANDREW NICKLIN, AND RUTH FADEN, PHD, MPH

Policymakers, researchers, and educators are now recognizing the long-term impacts of the COVID-19 pandemic on the well-being of children. Globally, an unprecedented 1.6 billion students experienced disruption in their education at some point in 2020 (Azevedo 2020). In the United States, approximately 3 million students may have completely disengaged from any type of formal education during the first seven months of the pandemic (Korman et al. 2020).

From March 2020 to May 11, 2023, when the US government declared an end to the public health emergency for COVID-19, the pandemic wreaked havoc on the United States education system, especially for students in kindergarten (K) through grade 12. While school closures were part of initial widespread public health measures to curb the pandemic, they were not without unintended short- and long-term consequences for children, even more so for children who already faced disparities in educational access and opportunities before the pandemic began (US Department of Education [DOE] 2021a). As the enormity of the suffering caused by the pandemic comes into fuller view, the educational impact on children will likely emerge as among the most dramatic and long-lasting (Faden 2020; Dorn et al. 2020; Fox et al. 2021; Kuhfeld et al. 2020).

The objectives of this chapter are

1. to discuss the impact of COVID-19 education disruptions on child well-being;
2. to highlight equity issues related to K–12 school responses; and
3. to describe the work of an interdisciplinary partnership, the Johns Hopkins eSchool+ Initiative, to bring attention to ethics and educational equity issues throughout the pandemic.

Timeline of COVID-19 School Closures and Education Policy Decisions

Schools across the United States began to close in early March 2020 (*Education Week* 2020b). By the end of March, more than 50 million school-age children across the United States had been impacted by school closures (see table 9.1). Wyoming and Montana were the only two states to reopen schools for in-person instruction during spring 2020; many states kept their school buildings shuttered and pursued various approaches to remote learning for the remainder of the 2019–2020 academic year (Ferren 2021; Dorn et al. 2020; Gross and Opalka 2020; Hough 2021).

The school closures in spring 2020 were abrupt and their duration uncertain. Contributing to the challenge of making decisions about when to reopen schools was the evolving situation with the pandemic, including considerable uncertainty about the role of schools in disease transmission and the risk of severe disease for children. Furthermore, early in the pandemic, there was limited testing capacity, and no COVID-19 vaccines or effective treatments were widely available.

During summer 2020, as information from the United Kingdom, Germany, and Israel began to shed light on COVID-19 transmission in schools, data also began to emerge about the negative effects of learning disruptions. In response, many leading authorities emphasized the urgency of reopening schools by fall 2020, especially given the disparate negative impact on students from disadvantaged backgrounds (Dorn et al. 2020; Nuzzo and Sharfstein 2020; Sharfstein and Morphew 2020). Despite the initial push to reopen schools in fall 2020, challenges persisted as the Trump administration and the US Department of Education pushed for school reopenings without providing clear guidance on how to do so safely.

At the same time, leading teacher unions threatened to strike unless appropriate measures were implemented to ensure the safety of educators and students (Black and Sciarra 2020; Perez 2020; Strauss 2020).

Against this political backdrop, state departments of education began to develop individual plans around how to reopen schools in fall 2020, including contingencies for remote support, should reopening schools for in-person instruction not be possible. These plans included discussions of *operational issues*, such as offering students Wi-Fi routers for remote learning or making provisions for to-go meal distribution when schools were closed, and *equity-focused considerations*, including the infrastructure needed to support students with special learning needs or disabilities, and establishing remote learning programs for parents who opted out of in-person learning for their children.

Despite hopes in summer 2020 that children could return to school buildings, many of the schools in the United States remained closed for in-person instruction during the first half of the 2020 to 2021 academic year, offering virtual or hybrid instruction (*Education Week* 2020a). This was due to a variety of factors, including limited and sometimes conflicting local, state, and federal guidance about how to reopen school buildings safely. Not surprisingly, there were marked regional variations, with more schools open for in-person instruction in states with Republican governors than Democratic governors (Lehrer-Small 2021). Some school systems that opened for in-person instruction were forced to close within weeks of opening due to COVID-19 outbreaks, highlighting the early challenges of what was a tumultuous year in K–12 education across the country (Hobbs 2020).

When President Biden was inaugurated in January 2021, he pledged to reopen K–12 schools for in-person instruction within his first one hundred days in office (Biden 2021). The push to reopen schools was aided by the US Food and Drug Administration (FDA) emergency use authorization (EUA) of the Pfizer-BioNTech COVID-19 vaccine in December 2020, followed shortly by the Moderna emergency use authorization, and by the president's urging, in March 2021, for states to prioritize vaccination of teachers and school staff (FDA 2024; Biden 2021).

Spring 2021 saw a return to in-person schooling for millions of students with frequently updated and sometimes conflicting Centers for Disease Control and Prevention (CDC) guidance (CDC 2021b). Even with more in-person schooling, several factors contributed to the continued disruption of education in spring 2021. These included limited access to COVID-19 vaccines for teachers, limited access to COVID-19 testing for the entire school community, and concerns from some teachers' unions and parent groups about the capacity and resources of schools needed to safely implement risk mitigation measures and keep students and teachers healthy. Some of these concerns were partially addressed by the American Rescue Plan (ARP) Elementary and Secondary School Emergency Relief Fund and President Biden's announcement of the COVID-19 vaccinations mandate for federal employees and those working in organizations with more than one hundred employees by fall 2021, although this mandate was later overturned (The White House 2021; US Department of Education 2021a).

By fall 2021, with more clarity in guidance from the CDC and ARP funding to implement safety measures, such as improved ventilation, many school districts were able to offer full or partial in-person instruction. And yet thousands of schools continued to experience intermittent disruptions to in-person learning, sometimes related to teacher shortages or fatigue and masking or vaccination disputes (Burbio 2021).

While the pandemic continued to ebb and flow, there are three indisputable facts. First, the United States education system was confronted with unprecedented challenges that forced rethinking how education is delivered for K–12 students. Second, COVID-19 educational disruptions harmed students broadly. Lastly, while millions of students were negatively impacted during the pandemic, those who were struggling before the pandemic were impacted more than others, creating the foundation for a generational effect that has widened existing inequities for children who are members of minoritized racial and ethnic groups and those living in communities with concentrated poverty. The COVID-19 pandemic exacerbated the existing precarity of housing, employment, food security, and education for these youth.

The Magnitude of Disadvantaged Students Impacted by the Pandemic

There are over 50 million children in grades K–12 across the United States (NCES 2020c). As school systems struggled to support student learning and well-being during the pandemic, specific groups of disadvantaged students were particularly susceptible to educational disruptions. These include the nearly one in five children living in poverty, one in seven qualifying for learning support under the Individuals with Disabilities Education Act, one in ten who are English Language Learners, and one in two public school students who are eligible for free and reduced-price meals (Kids Count Data Center 2020; NCES 2020a; NCES 2020b; NCES 2021b).

While these numbers start to portray the enormity of students who were at risk during the pandemic, there are additional groups that newly qualified as at risk due to the pandemic. These include children whose parents were essential workers, those living in multigenerational households, and children without access to devices or stable Internet to enable remote learning. Students with preexisting health problems were another group at risk for disproportionate impact during the pandemic. Some students qualified for their school's home and hospital program and were learning from home before the pandemic, while others newly qualified due to comorbidities that increased the risk of contracting COVID-19 or developing severe disease. Developing a broad understanding of all the at-risk groups, which sometimes overlap, was the key to fully understanding and responding to the widening educational inequities created by the pandemic (*Education Week* 2021; NCES 2018b; Pilkauskas et al. 2020; Rothstein and Olympia 2020).

COVID-19's Impact on School Support Systems

Schools are not only instrumental for a child's education, but they also frequently play a critical role in the provision of meals, health services, safety, supervision, and shelter. For students to succeed in school, these additional social supports are vital to their academic achievement and health. The recognition of the inter-relatedness of learning and health is informed by the CDC Whole School, Whole Child, Whole Community model (CDC 2021f). For many children, these school-based services are essential, as schools may provide the only outlet to receive needed services and resources.

As schools are a critical link to the provision of many school-based supports and services, children were at increased risk early in the pandemic when school buildings were closed. Early school responses focused mainly on learning and food provision, with significantly less attention to providing other essential services. After three school years were disrupted by the pandemic, an accumulating body of data has documented the deleterious impacts of such loss of school-based support services (Annie E. Casey Foundation 2020; Garcia-Area and D'Souza 2020; Jackson and Bowdon 2020).

Provision of meals. More than 20 million children rely on schools to provide breakfast or lunch (Bauer 2020a, 2020b). Surveys indicate that one in five mothers with children younger than twelve years old reported their children going hungry during the pandemic, with rates three to four times higher among Black and Hispanic households (Bauer 2020a, 2020b). Prior to the pandemic, one in two public school students were eligible for free and reduced-price meals at school (NCES 2020b).

During the height of the pandemic, with the closure of school buildings and stay-at-home orders, children lost access to these daily sources of meals. From May 2020 to September 2021, children missed a collective 1 billion school meals, with major urban districts all reporting a drop in children accessing meals, even when schools made contingencies for food distribution when school buildings were closed (McLoughlin et al. 2020; Rothstein and Olympia 2020). Whether these children accessed nutrition via other means is unknown; however, there can be long-term health and development impacts from even short periods of food insecurity (Zippel and Sherman 2021).

Provision of health services. Before the pandemic, schools routinely provided a range of health services for students, including screenings for vision and hearing, preventive care, and immunizations through school-based health centers (SBHCs), and additional vision, dental, and mental and behavioral health services through partnerships with external providers (Vision for Baltimore 2020). This was especially critical given children in medically underserved communities have higher rates of asthma, obesity, and mental health disorders and are less likely to receive routine care from community providers (H. E. Love et al. 2019). During school building closures, many students did not access health services previously received in the school setting or even in the community. For example, there was a 21.5 percent decrease in immunizations for children aged eighteen or younger as compared to prior years (Bramer et al. 2020). Reports indicated cessations and delays in routine screening programs, such as vision screenings (Antonio Aguirre et al. 2021). At the same time, there was an exponential increase in mental health symptoms reported among children (Burke et al. 2021; Gupta and Jawanda 2020; Kranz et al. 2022).

As schools reopened and pivoted toward recovery efforts, school nurses, school health suites, and SBHCs faced a surge in demand due to delayed care. At the time, they were called upon to provide an array of COVID-19 services, including case management, testing, and vaccination for eligible students and teachers, risking further stress to an already over-taxed system (Lesser et al. 2021; Miller 2021).

Safety/supervision during the school day. Another notable challenge without regular in-person teacher contact relates to the teachers' role in identifying children in high-risk social situations. Teachers and other school personnel are one group fundamental in recognizing suspected child abuse. In 2018, teachers and other school personnel reported one-fifth of suspected child abuse cases, surpassing the number of reports made by law enforcement, medical professionals, and social workers individually (Baron et al. 2020). Early in the pandemic, when schools were closed, reports of suspected child abuse dropped by 25 percent in Arizona, according to the Arizona Department of Child Safety (Baron et al. 2020). However, there were concerns of more severe cases of child abuse than before the pandemic, suggesting that many cases were going undetected (Weiner et al. 2020).

Shelter. Even before the pandemic, thousands of children were experiencing homelessness or unstable housing situations. School buildings offered a place of shelter during the school day and are often supplemented by before- or after-school programs. As of February 2021, more than 5 million households with children were behind on rent payments, with almost half of these reporting a likelihood of needing to leave their home within sixty days (Todres and Meeler 2021). Children without secure housing faced immense challenges during the pandemic, and yet providing additional support for children with transient housing situations was often not addressed by schools or state reopening plans, being discussed in only 25 percent of school reopening plans, according to one analysis (Li et al. 2020).

Examining School Closures through an Equity Lens: The eSchool+ Initiative

On February 20, 2020, after a CDC official raised the possibility that schools might close in the United States due to the looming pandemic, Dr. Ruth Faden, a bioethicist and founder of the Berman Institute of Bioethics, published an op-ed piece in the *Baltimore Sun*. She warned, "As in all public health emergencies, poor children and poor families will suffer the most." Dr. Faden called for developing COVID-19 policies that not only met the bar of public health necessity but also included "active measures to mitigate the disproportionate burden that will fall on our most vulnerable children" (Faden 2020).

In response to this call to action, the eSchool+ Initiative was established as an interdisciplinary partnership to contribute to a safe and healthy return to quality schooling for all the world's students, particularly those who suffered disproportionately during the pandemic because of systemic disadvantage. The eSchool+ Initiative included broad representation from the Johns Hopkins University Schools of Education, Public Health, and Medicine; the Berman Institute of Bioethics; and the Center for Civic Impact, bringing expertise in ethics, equity, structural injustice, education, school health, food security, public health, public policy, and data visualization. Beginning in March 2020, the eSchool+ Initiative developed a suite of data trackers, position papers, and guidance documents to assist policymakers, educators, and public health professionals in critical decision-

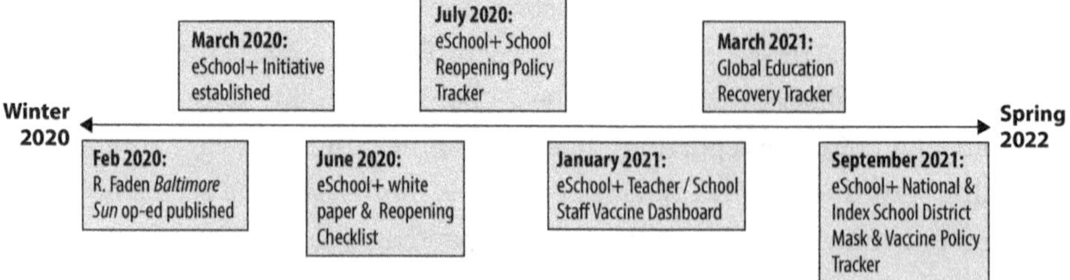

Figure 9.1 Timeline of eSchool+ Initiative development of resources for decision-making about K–12 school closings and reopenings around the world.

making for K–12 school closing and reopening, both nationally and globally (figure 9.1).

The Ethics of School Reopening

Early in the pandemic, during the spring and summer of 2020, the collaborators of the eSchool+ Initiative recognized that how to reopen schools was one of the most pressing decisions facing political leaders across the country. One of the primary ethical challenges for decision-makers was determining how to balance the interests of children and the interests of society in the context of evolving uncertainties and policy responses that risked exacerbating existing inequities.

Although there was concern about multisystem inflammatory syndrome and long COVID, the case remained that school-age children rarely die or become seriously ill from COVID-19 (CDC 2021d). However, all children were being severely impacted by school closures, disadvantaged children most of all. The burden on children was particularly ethically unsettling amid many uncertainties. What children lose by not being in school is enormous; school attendance is a life-defining experience critical for educational, social, and emotional development. However, most school districts in the United States were forced to offer hybrid or remote learning options when access to school buildings became limited due to concerns about COVID-19 community transmission. Even now, we do not fully know the effects—academically, developmentally, or emotionally—that remote and hybrid experiences provided compared to typical in-person instruction. Furthermore, many students, most likely systematically disadvantaged students, were never able to access alternate modes of instruction due to digital and/or economic divides, thereby increasing the already glaring educational gap between students (Korman et al. 2020).

The eSchool+ COVID-19 School Reopening Checklist

The eSchool+ COVID-19 School Reopening Checklist, released in late spring 2020, provided guidance for schools, district leaders, and other key stakeholders in navigating the complex considerations required to make decisions about opening and closing schools in the last months of the 2019–20 school year, as well as the entirety of the 2020–21 academic year. The checklist facilitated the systematic assessment of needs and resources for reopening in six areas: continuity of learning, infection control and facilities, food security, health, housing and safety, and supervision, while also emphasizing areas requiring attention from an equity and ethics perspective (table 9.2).

US School Reopening Policy Tracker (2020–21)

The eSchool+ US School Reopening Policy Tracker (SRT), which launched in July 2020, provided detailed information about school reopening plans for the 2020–21 academic year in fifty-seven jurisdictions (fifty states, five territories, the District of Columbia, and the Bureau of Indian Education) (figure 9.2). The SRT included publicly available information, collected and visualized on a website in real time, about whether each of these plans addressed six operational and six ethics and equity criteria (table 9.3). The operational criteria addressed practical hurdles (e.g., spacing of desks, seating on school buses) that would need to be cleared to safely resume in-person instruction in the context of an ongoing pandemic. The ethics and equity criteria highlighted crucial considerations to address in reopening plans to minimize the negative impact on disadvantaged students. For example, the tracker monitored whether state reopening plans included provisions for remote learning and distribution of devices / Wi-Fi hotspots, as well as whether there were plans to support students living in unstable/transient housing.

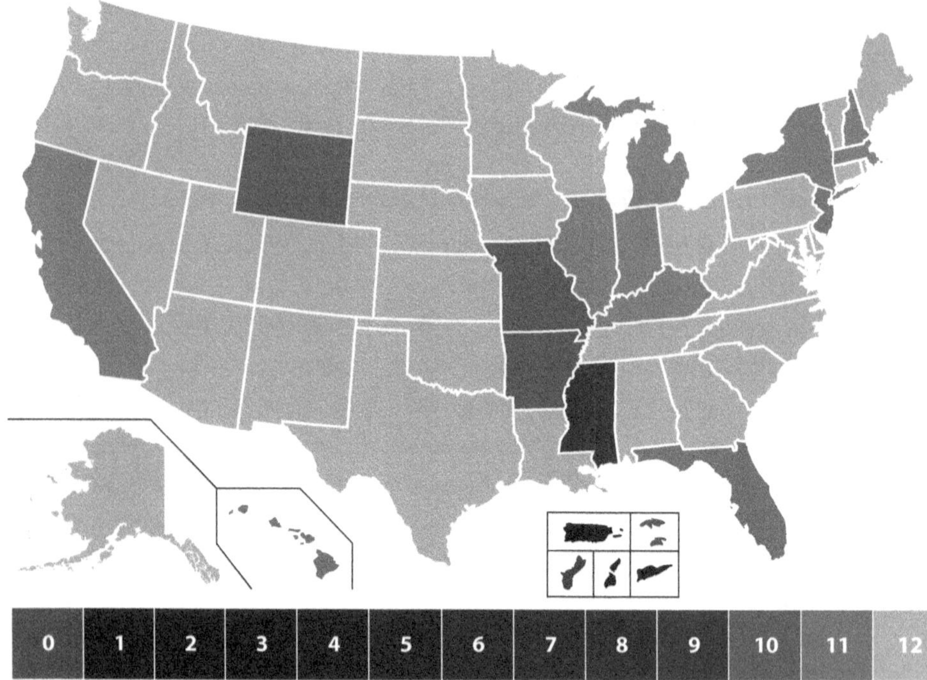

Number of categories included in state reopening plan

1. Core Academics
2. SARS CoV-2 Protection
3. Before- & After-School Programs
4. School Access & Transportation
5. Student Health Services
6. Food & Nutrition
7. Parent Choice
8. Teacher & Staff Choice
9. Children of Poverty and Systemic Disadvantage
10. Children with Special Needs / ESL / Gifted and Twice Exceptional
11. Privacy
12. Engagement & Transparency

Figure 9.2 2021 map depicting operational and ethical categories considered in US state/territory pandemic-era reopening plans.
Source: Redrawn from https://equityschoolplus.jhu.edu/reopening-policy-tracker/

At its launch, the SRT filled a significant need for comprehensive and reliable information about K–12 reopening plans and received more than 168,000 website visits within its first few weeks. Designed to inform decision-making about the 2020–21 school year, the information curated on the SRT was intended for use by education and public health policy stakeholders and researchers, teachers, and school staff from across the United States, as well as parents, child advocates, journalists, and edu-

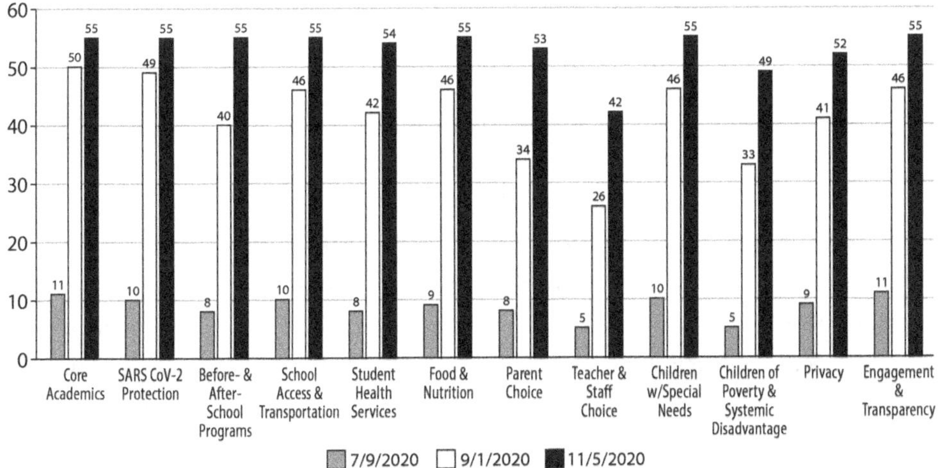

Figure 9.3 Time-trend analysis of operational and equity considerations in 2020–21 school reopening plans.
Source: Data drawn from https://equityschoolplus.jhu.edu/reopening-policy-tracker/

cation researchers. By using a public-facing data initiative, the eSchool+ Initiative also hoped that deficiencies in equity categories would serve as a call to action for allocating resources to support those impacted the most.

A time-trend analysis from July to November 2020 showed that school reopening plans were initially more likely to address operational categories than equity considerations, although there were positive trends for both categories over time (figure 9.3). While a causal relationship between the SRT and updates to state reopening plans cannot definitively be established, it is worth noting that multiple media outlets covered stories about the SRT and used the tracker to compare their state plans with others. Teacher and staff choice about returning to in-person schooling, support for children of systemic disadvantage, and privacy issues remained the most frequently neglected categories. These findings were corroborated by an analysis by Li et al., who also reported marked variation in state-level guidance about reopening K–12 schools, especially for the students "most vulnerable to learning loss or reduced access to basic needs" (Li et al. 2020, 38).

Teacher and School Staff COVID-19 Vaccination Dashboard

When Moderna and Pfizer COVID-19 vaccines received EUA status for adults from the Food and Drug Administration in late 2020, the eSchool+ team recognized how pivotal teachers' COVID-19 vaccine access would be to schools returning fully to in-person learning. Leading policy organizations deliberated about where teachers and school staff fit into vaccine allocation frameworks. The National Academies of Sciences, Engineering, and Medicine included teachers and school staff in Phase 2 of a four-phased plan vaccine rollout directly after Phase 1: older adults, immunocompromised individuals, and essential workers (Gayle et al. 2020). The Advisory Committee on Immunization Practices, which released recommendations in December 2020, categorized teachers as "frontline essential workers" and included them in Phase 1b of their two-phased plan (Phase 1 was divided into groups a, b, and c), along with first responders and public transit workers, among others (Dooling 2020).

The eSchool+ Teacher and School Staff COVID-19 Vaccination Dashboard launched in winter 2021 as the national conversation focused on vaccine access for teachers. The purpose of the dashboard was to capture real-time information about the phases of vaccine rollout in fifty-seven jurisdictions (fifty states, five territories, the District of Columbia, and the Bureau of Indian Education) and how each jurisdiction prioritized teachers and other school staff in their vaccine allocation plans (figure 9.4). In January 2021, when vaccine availability was still limited, fifty states and the District of Columbia had published their initial Phase 1 (highest priority) vaccination groups. Teachers and/or school staff were included in Phase 1 in twenty-three states. For twenty of twenty-three of these states, teachers/school staff were in Phase 1b. In one state, they were in Phase 1 without any subphases, and in two states they were in Phase 1d. Twenty-eight states included teachers in a later phase or did not discuss their prioritization at all (Crane et al. 2021).

While CDC recommendations issued in February 2021 did not require vaccination of teachers as a prerequisite for a return to in-person learning,

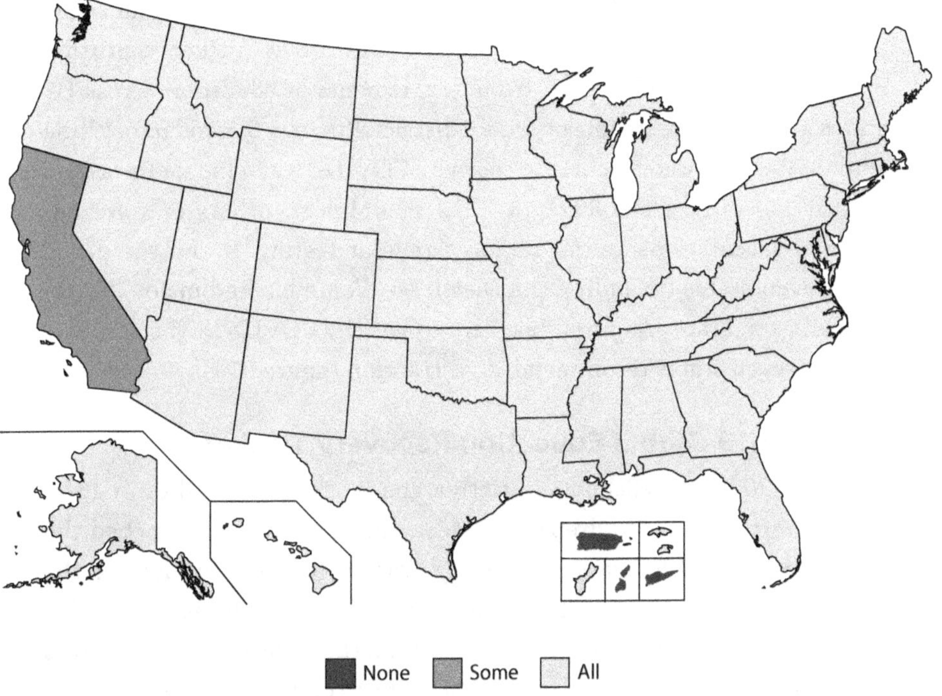

Figure 9.4 2021 Teacher and School Staff COVID-19 Vaccine Priority Group (States, Territories, and District of Columbia).
Source: Redrawn from https://equityschoolplus.jhu.edu/vaccinations-dashboard/

many education groups and teachers endorsed this view (CDC 2021c; Walker 2021). Both the American Federation of Teachers and the National Education Association (NEA) advocated for prioritizing educators to receive vaccines "because of the importance of safe, equitable, and effective in-person instruction and support" (NEA 2020, para. 4; Weingarten 2020). On March 2, 2021, the Biden administration released a directive instructing states to prioritize vaccination of pre-kindergarten to grade 12 teachers, staff, and childcare workers (Biden 2021). Before, thirty-five states (including the District of Columbia) had begun vaccinating teachers. After the directive, seventeen states expanded the eligibility of teachers. In three states, teacher eligibility was extended to all teachers statewide, whereas, in the remaining fourteen states, teachers became newly eligible.

In late 2021, eSchool+ launched the 2021 to 2022 National and Index School District Mask and COVID-19 Vaccine Policy Tracker, capturing mask and vaccine policy data from departments of education across US states and an index sample of school districts (figures 9.5 and 9.6). While some states required teachers to receive a COVID-19 vaccine for in-person instruction during the 2021 to 2022 school year, others only recommended vaccinations and/or required regular testing. In our sample of fifty-seven states (including the District of Columbia and major US territories), ten states required teachers to get the COVID-19 vaccine, and twenty-seven states recommended vaccination (figure 9.7).

COVID-19 Global Education Recovery Tracker

In March 2021, the eSchool+ Initiative, the World Bank, and United Nations International Children's Emergency Fund (UNICEF) launched the COVID-19 Global Education Recovery Tracker (G-ERT) to monitor the impact of COVID-19 on K–12, vocational, and higher education globally. The G-ERT captured publicly available data on the state of education across all grade levels, including in-person academic supports, remote learning modalities, and teacher prioritization for COVID-19 vaccines. The data displayed on a publicly available website were intended to support educators, policymakers, and researchers as the conversations pivoted from the emergency-oriented educational response to recovery efforts in 2022 and beyond (figures 9.8 and 9.9).

Mask Requirements for Teachers and Students during the 2021–22 Academic Year

Early on, recommendations by experts about the role of masks for students or teachers in a safe return to school were not always clear or consistent. In summer 2021, the CDC initially indicated masks were not required and later reversed this recommendation, while the American Academy of Pediatrics (AAP) endorsed universal masking, and school districts bemoaned another year without clear guidance from authorities (CDC 2021e; American Academy of Pediatrics 2021; Balingit et al. 2021). In fall 2021, the surge of the Delta variant and its concerning implications for child health

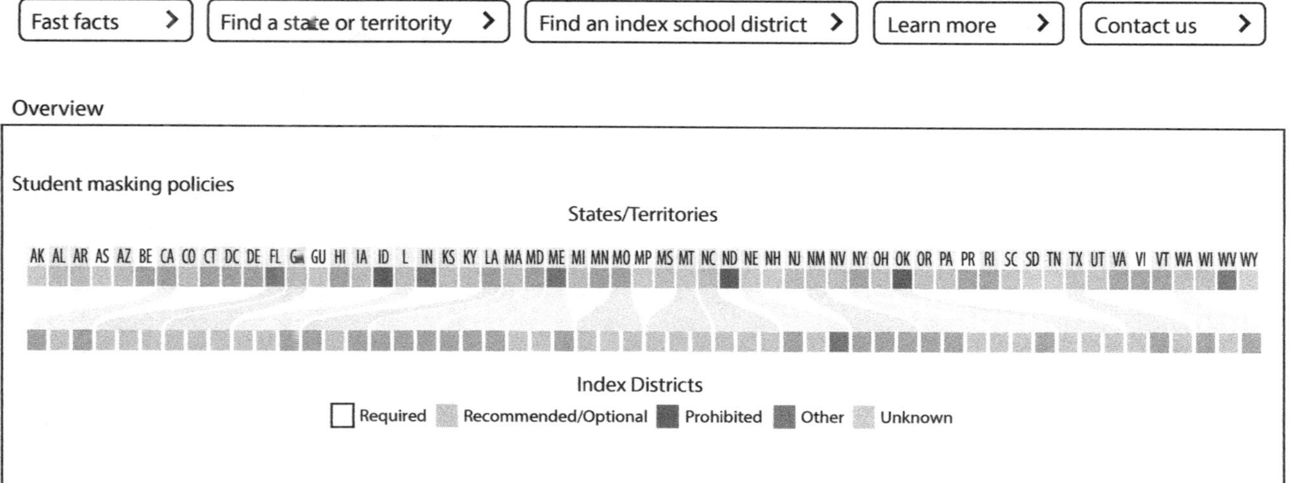

Figure 9.5 Screenshot of Johns Hopkins University (2021) National and Index School District Mask & COVID-19 Vaccine Policy Tracker.
Source: https://equityschool.plus/national-and-index-district-school-tracker/

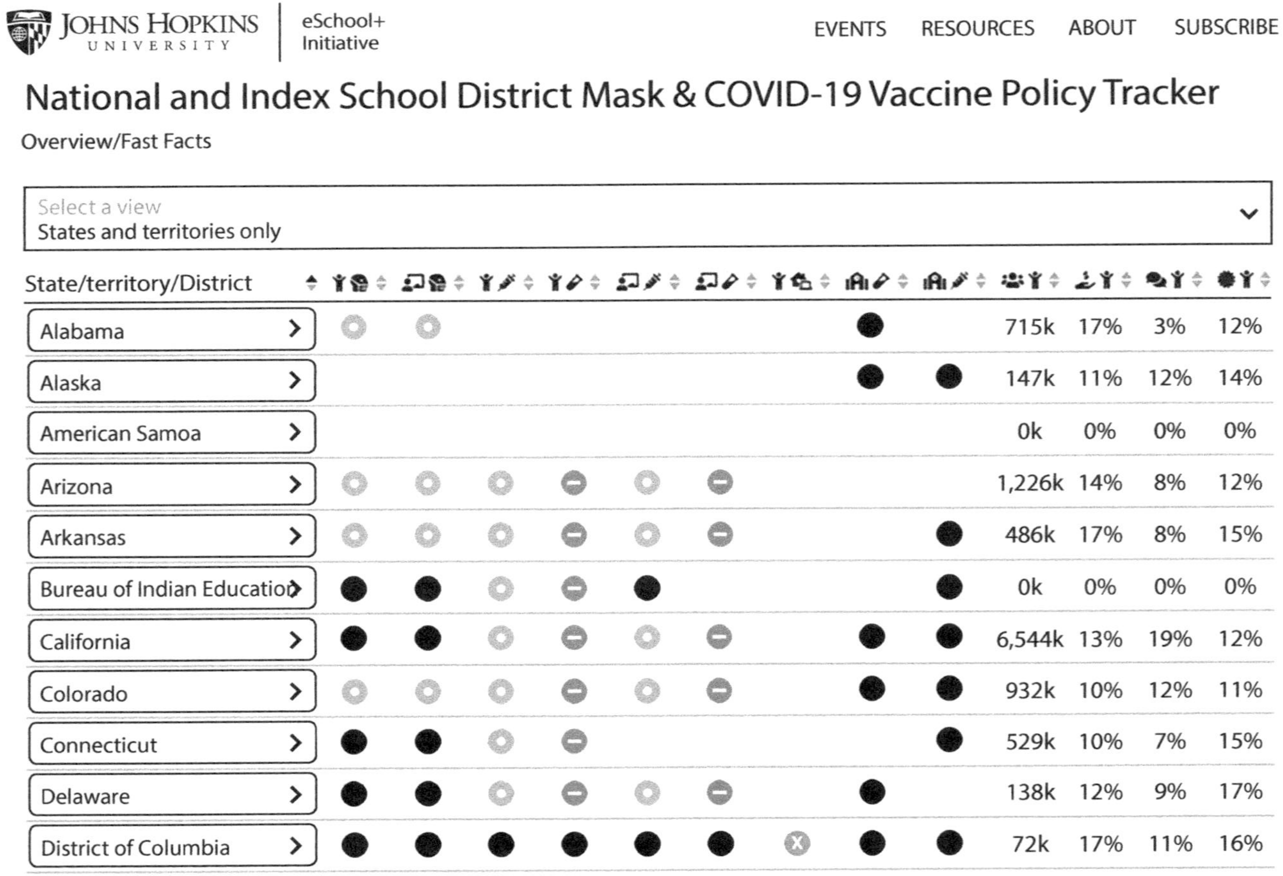

JOHNS HOPKINS UNIVERSITY | eSchool+ Initiative

EVENTS RESOURCES ABOUT SUBSCRIBE

National and Index School District Mask & COVID-19 Vaccine Policy Tracker

Overview/Fast Facts

Select a view
States and territories only

State/territory/District													
Alabama	○	○						●		715k	17%	3%	12%
Alaska								●	●	147k	11%	12%	14%
American Samoa										0k	0%	0%	0%
Arizona	○	○	○	⊖	○	⊖				1,226k	14%	8%	12%
Arkansas	○	○	○	⊖	○	⊖			●	486k	17%	8%	15%
Bureau of Indian Education	●	●	○	⊖	●				●	0k	0%	0%	0%
California	●	●	○	⊖	○	⊖		●	●	6,544k	13%	19%	12%
Colorado	○	○	○	⊖	○	⊖		●	●	932k	10%	12%	11%
Connecticut	●	●	○	⊖					●	529k	10%	7%	15%
Delaware	●	●	○	⊖	○	⊖		●		138k	12%	9%	17%
District of Columbia	●	●	●	●	●	●	⊗	●	●	72k	17%	11%	16%

Figure 9.6 Screenshot of Johns Hopkins University (2021) National and Index School District Mask & COVID-19 Vaccine Policy Tracker (states and territories only view).

Source: https://equityschool.plus/national-and-index-district-school-tracker/ [illegible]

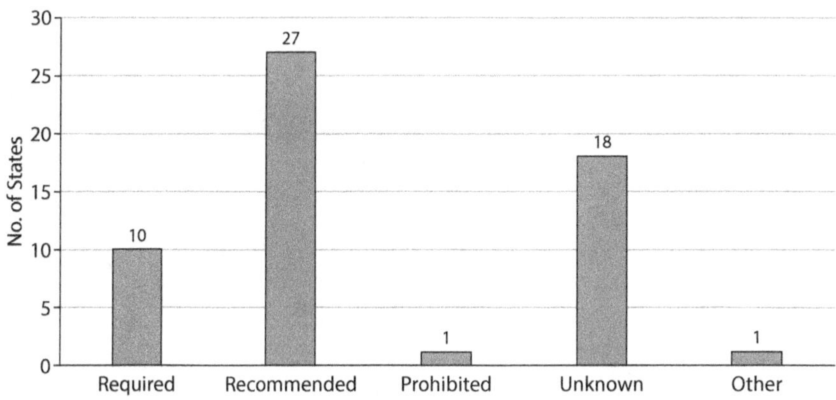

Figure 9.7 State COVID-19 vaccine mandates for teachers.
Source: Data drawn from https://equityschoolplus.jhu.edu/national-and-index-district-school-tracker/

complicated the situation further. Heated debates occurred about whether to implement a state or district-level mask mandate. At the same time, several states made moves to ban mask mandates. These conversations took on greater significance given there was an accumulating body of evidence about the benefits of in-person instruction for K–12 students and the deleterious effect of being out of school for students from disadvantaged backgrounds (Dorn et al. 2020).

In fall 2021, there was a near consensus among public health experts that mask requirements for both teachers, staff, and students were critical to the safe reopening of schools, yet there was still marked variation in policy positions adopted by state departments of education. The eSchool+ 2021 to 2022 National and Index School District Mask and COVID-19 Vaccine Policy Tracker captured this variation initially and trends over time.

In September 2021, of the fifty-six index school districts included, 75 percent (n = 42) required masks for teachers, staff, and students, and an additional 23 percent (n = 13) recommended masking. No districts prohibited the wearing of masks by both teachers, and staff or students. Of particular concern was that school districts serving the highest concentration of poor children in their states were initially the least likely to impose mask requirements. These were the districts whose children were most

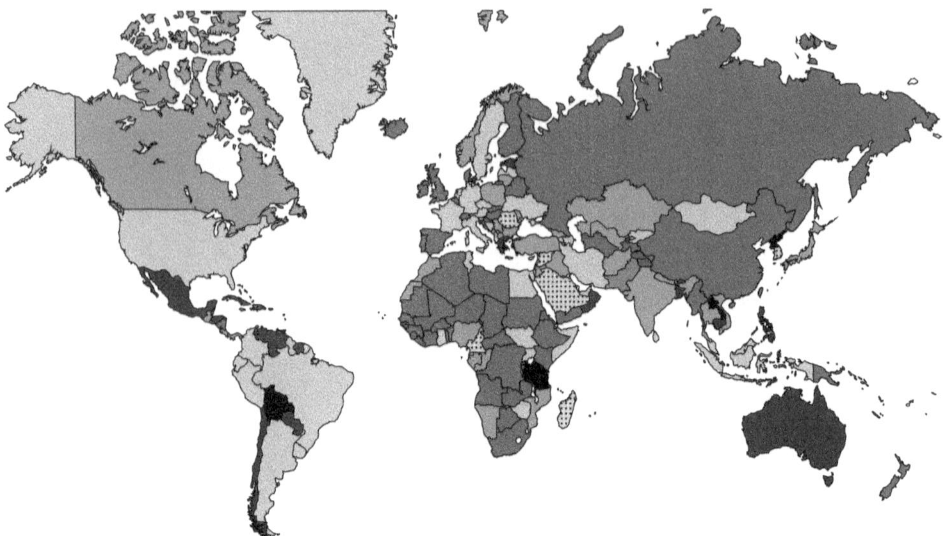

Legend
In-person education: Schools are open, and students have returned for in-person instruction.
Hybrid education: Schools are open, combining remote learning and in-person instruction.
Remote education: Schools are closed and students are exclusively learning remotely.
Mixed/multiple: Schools are operating with a combination of the following: in-person, hybrid, remote, and closed due to COVID-19.
Extended break: Schools are closed due to a regular school calendar closure (e.g., a holiday).
No instruction / closed due to COVID-19: Schools are closed due to COVID-19, and no education services are currently available.
Unknown / Data Not Available: Unable to obtain information through publicly available data.

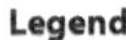

Figure 9.8 School status / education modality world map showing how education was provided in each country during COVID-19 pandemic.
Source: Redrawn from https://www.covideducationrecovery.global/data/

likely to have been out of school during the first year of the pandemic, who were at the greatest risk of learning loss, and who came from communities with higher rates of COVID morbidity and mortality (White et al. 2021; Kim et al. 2020). Parents from minorities or ethnic groups, who were over-represented in low-income communities, were more likely than White parents to be concerned about whether it was safe for their children to return to school; the absence of mask mandates may have reinforced these concerns (Gilbert et al. 2020).

States and districts varied in their masking policies over time, as well

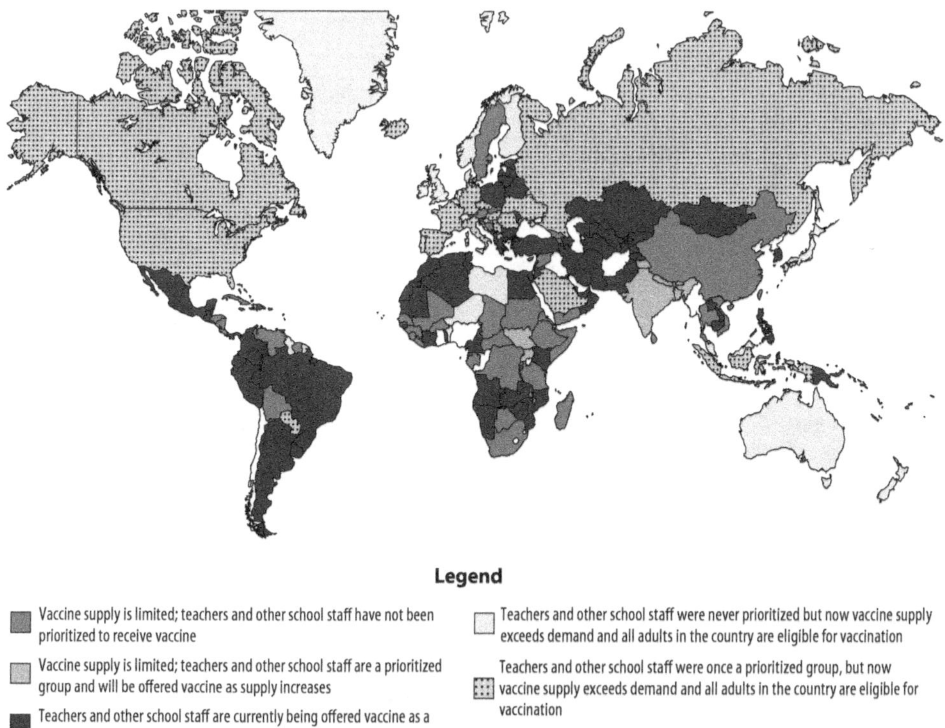

Figure 9.9 World map showing how different countries prioritized (or failed to prioritize) teachers and school staff for COVID-19 vaccines.
Source: Redrawn from https://www.covideducationrecovery.global/data/

as by the political affiliation of their governor (figures 9.10 and 9.11). Some masking guidance led to litigation; of the ten states that banned or brought legal dispute due to stricter mask guidance, 60 percent were blocked or overturned (Decker 2021). In March 2022, many mask mandates had been rescinded, yet as other variants arise and vaccines became available for people of all ages, the mask policies continued to change.

Even before the pandemic, existing structural injustices impacted the well-being of students. Irrefutably, COVID-19 and school disruptions (ranging from complete closures to periodic quarantines) have exacerbated systemic inequities and injustices and harmed child well-being.

The pandemic resulted in three waves of inequity for disadvantaged

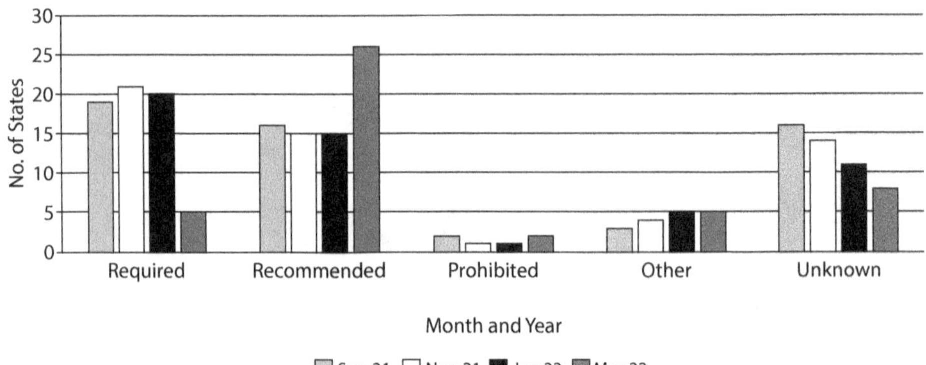

Figure 9.10 State Department of Education student masking policies during the 2021 to 2022 school year.
Source: Data drawn from eSchool+ National and Index School District Mask & COVID-19 Vaccine Policy Tracker at https://equityschoolplus.jhu.edu/national-and-index-district-school-tracker/

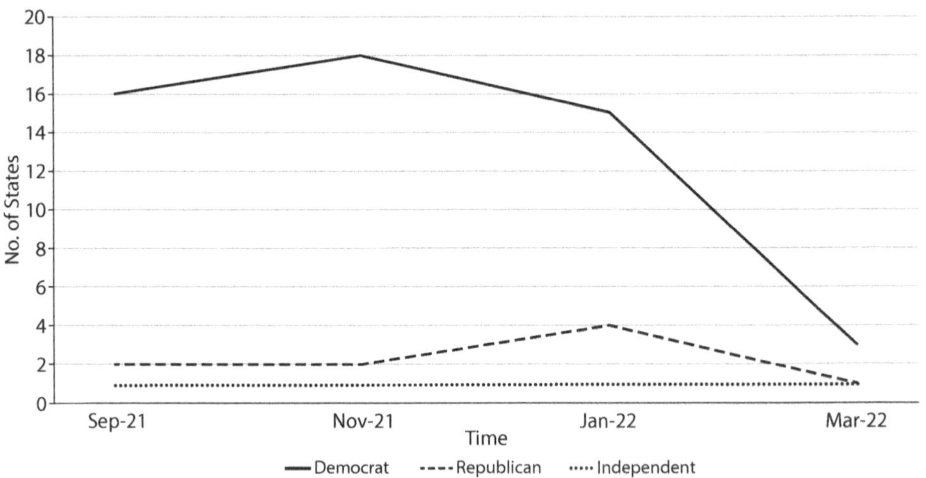

Figure 9.11 Student mask mandates by political party of governor during the 2021 to 2022 school year.
Source: Data drawn from eSchool+ National and Index School District Mask & COVID-19 Vaccine Policy Tracker at https://equityschoolplus.jhu.edu/national-and-index-district-school-tracker/

children. During the first wave (spring 2020), children experienced higher absenteeism rates, limited access to technology, and a lack of formal instruction plans. During the 2020–21 school year, gaps in access to technology remained, and chronic absenteeism, learning loss, and mental health issues continued to have a disproportionate impact. In 2022 to 2023 and beyond, there are risks of further and compounded negative impacts on grade attrition, performance on standardized assessments, high school graduation rates, future employment, and health.

Key Points from the COVID-19 Pandemic

1. The COVID-19 pandemic highlighted the deleterious effects school closures can have on a child's well-being and future.
2. Students, especially from minoritized racial and ethnic groups and poor students, experienced the greatest negative impact of the pandemic.
3. Schools play a vital role in (1) provision of meals, (2) provision of health services, (3) safety/supervision, and (4) shelter, in addition to education to students. All these support systems were disrupted during the pandemic, impacting children's well-being.
4. The eSchool+ Initiative was an example of a multidisciplinary partnership focused on data collection, visualization, and guidance

Table 9.1 United States K–12 Education Disruption Timeline Due to COVID-19

March 2020	K–12 schools close across the United States
Spring 2020	K–12 schools partially reopen, mostly with remote learning options
Summer 2020	State Boards of Education begin releasing 2020–2021 academic year school reopening plans
August 2020	K–12 schools begin to reopen (in-person, virtual, and/or hybrid)
January 2021	President Joe Biden announces plan to reopen schools during the first 100 days of the new administration
March 2021	President Biden announces prioritization of teachers and school staff for COVID-19 vaccines

Table 9.2 The eSchool+ COVID-19 School Reopening Checklist

Continuity of Learning	How many students have been out of contact with teachers or school administration for some or most of the closure? What were the primary methods of record-keeping for missing students? How many or what percentage of students were chronically absent during the COVID-19 school closure? How many students continued learning with packets only? How many students are at risk of dropout or in need of academic interventions for progression? How many students reside in areas where broadband access is limited? How many students are ELL (English language learners)? How many students have learning or other disabilities that require accommodations in the school setting?
Engagement	What ways have students been engaged in decisions about reopening? • What percentage of students have been engaged in the decisions about reopening?
Food Security	How many students are eligible for direct certification, FARMS (free and reduced meals), and/or are economically disadvantaged? What percentage of students participated in food giveaways or meal distributions? • Are there students newly eligible for FARMS or direct certification?
Health	What percentage of students regularly interact with the health office on a routine basis (e.g., medication administration)? How many students routinely receive somatic or behavioral health services in the school setting? Have these students received any school-based health services during the school closure? How many students reside in a dwelling where an occupant has been diagnosed with COVID-19? What proportion of students live in zip codes with high caseloads of COVID-19? • How many students required home learning services for a health or other reason before schools were closed?

Supervision	How many students have parents who are essential workers? What plans have parents put in place to provide for supervision if they are essential workers? • Have schools prioritized these students for outreach to evaluate their supervision circumstances?
Housing/Safety	How many students are experiencing homelessness or otherwise considered unstably housed? How many students are at risk of becoming homeless because of familial job losses? How many students cannot be currently located? Will this affect their ability to reliably get to school? Is there a way to get updated addresses for these students? How many students live in households with individuals at higher risk of contracting COVID-19? For example, with older adults (e.g., grandparents) or other individuals with chronic health conditions (e.g., heart or lung conditions, cancer).

for education stakeholders and policymakers, with the mission to bring attention to the importance of ethics and equity considerations related to school disruptions.

Conclusion

The educational system faced an enormous challenge of mitigating the damages and continued risks of harm that all children, but especially systematically disadvantaged children, experienced from this pandemic. Schools responded by building new capacities, using technology, and increasing engagement with families to help children and support social needs. The inequities laid bare by the pandemic received national attention at the time and continue to do so even several years later. There is a strong case for reimagining a better education system. Looking ahead and planning for future pandemics, should they arise, it is imperative to have plans for adopting new technologies, approaches, and remedies for the adverse effects of pandemic disruptions on the well-being of children.

Table 9.3 US School Reopening Tracker Classification Scheme

Type	Subcategories	Components
Operational	**Core Academics**	• Instruction (in-class, distance, hybrid) • Schedules and learning time • Instructional interventions • Physical, health education; socio-emotional learning • Enrichment, electives, externships • Assessments and accountability • Internet connectivity • Children with different priority needs • School staffing, certification, and professional development
	SARS CoV-2 Protection	• PPE requirements • Hygiene and sanitization • Screening and COVID-19 testing protocols • Environmental services staff • Physical environment; restructuring classrooms and public spaces • Student flow and movement
	Before-/After-School Programs	• Childcare • Athletics or extracurricular/clubs
	Building Access & Student Transportation	• School bus cleaning and infection control protocol • Public transportation safety • School entrance and exit route
	School Health Services	• Annual school health requirements • School-based health services • School nurse health suite
	Food and Nutrition	• Meal provision during in-person learning • Meal provision during partial or full remote learning time

Equity	**Parent Choice**	• Parental requests for in-person or distance instruction • Child and family best interests
	Teacher and Other School Personnel Choice	• Staff options for returning to work • Qualification factors for in-person/remote options • Teachers/other professional staff at increased risk/concern for COVID-19 • Support staff (food service, sanitation, etc.) at increased risk/concern for COVID-19 • Teacher/other professional staff/family not at increased risk, but other personal reasons • Support staff/family not at increased risk, but other personal reasons
	Children with Special Needs/IEP/ESL/Gifted & Twice Exceptional	• Support services • Learning accommodations • Transportation • Staffing and scheduling
	Children of Poverty, Color, Systematic Disadvantage. Low-Income Parents & Parents Who Are Essential Workers	• Provisions to lessen disproportionate negative impact from school disruptions • Students experiencing homelessness • Students in foster care • Students in juvenile detention facilities • Students eligible for free and reduced meals (FARMs)/children living in high-poverty neighborhoods, low-income families • Children of color • Immigrant families • Ongoing assessment of extent of disproportionate impact on these groups
	Privacy	• COVID-19 screening, testing, and tracing • Telemedicine • Requirements for staff/students' disclosure of personal health information that may impact choices around returning to school due to risk of COVID
	Engagement and Transparency about COVID and School Closures/Reopening	• Process for engaging stakeholders in development of policy/guidance about school response • COVID-19 parent/student/staff health education • Ongoing engagement strategies as COVID-19 experiences proceeds through the school year

Contributors

Christopher Morphew, PhD, is the dean of Johns Hopkins University's School of Education, where he is also a professor. He is the coeditor of *The Challenge of Independent Colleges: Moving Research to Practice* and *Privatizing the Public University: Perspectives from across the Academy.*

Vanya C. Jones, PhD, MPH, is the assistant dean for community-engaged research and an associate professor of health, behavior, and society at the Johns Hopkins Bloomberg School of Public Health. She is also the associate director of the Johns Hopkins Urban Health Institute.

Ashley E. Cureton, PhD, MSW, is an assistant professor in the School of Social Work and the Marsal Family School of Education at the University of Michigan.

Annette Campbell Anderson, PhD, MSEd, MPP, is an assistant professor at Johns Hopkins University's School of Education, where she is also the deputy director of the Center for Safe & Healthy Schools and the curriculum director of the Johns Hopkins HEAT Corps.

Megan Collins, MD, MPH, is the Allan and Claire Jensen Professor of Ophthalmology at Johns Hopkins University, where she is an associate professor within the School of Medicine's Wilmer Eye Institute and the director of the Johns Hopkins Consortium for School-Based Health Solutions, which she cofounded.

Ruth Faden, PhD, MPH, the founder of the Johns Hopkins Berman Institute of Bioethics, is the Philip Franklin Wagley Professor of Biomedical Ethics and a professor of health policy and management at Johns Hopkins University.

Ashley A. Grant, PhD, is a senior researcher in the School of Education at Johns Hopkins University.

Sheldon F. Greenberg, PhD, is Professor Emeritus at Johns Hopkins University's School of Education and a senior faculty associate at the Johns Hopkins Bloomberg School of Public Health.

Odis Johnson Jr., PhD, is a Bloomberg Distinguished Professor at Johns Hopkins University's School of Education. He is also the social policy and STEM equity executive director at the Johns Hopkins Center for Safe & Healthy Schools and the director of Hopkins's Institute in Critical Quantitative, Computational, and Mixed Methodologies.

Sara Johnson, PhD, MPH, is the Blanket Fort Foundation Professor in Pediatric Population Health and Health Equity Research at Johns Hopkins University, where she is also a professor of pediatrics within the School of Medicine.

Jonathan M. Links, PhD, is the vice provost and chief risk officer at Johns Hopkins University, is where he is a professor in the Schools of Public Health, Medicine, Education, Engineering, and Business.

Richard Lofton Jr., PhD, is an assistant professor at Johns Hopkins University's School of Education.

Douglas J. Mac Iver, PhD, is a research professor at Johns Hopkins University's School of Education, where he is the codirector of the Center for Social Organization of Schools.

Olivia Marcucci, PhD, is an assistant professor at Johns Hopkins University's School of Education.

Beth Marshall, DrPH, MPH, is an associate practice professor of population, family, and reproductive health at the Johns Hopkins Bloomberg School of Public Health, where she is the associate director of the Center for Adolescent Health.

Andrew Nicklin is a senior research data manager at Johns Hopkins University's Bloomberg Center for Government Excellence.

Asari Offiong, PhD, MPH, is a senior research scientist of sexual and reproductive health at Child Trends.

Terrinieka W. Powell, PhD, MA, is the vice chair of inclusion, diversity, anti-racism and equity (IDARE) and an associate professor of population, family, and reproductive health at the Johns Hopkins Bloomberg School of Public Health. She is also the associate director of the Center for Adolescent Health.

Alan Regenberg, MBe, is the director of outreach and research support at the Johns Hopkins Berman Institute of Bioethics.

Chris Swanson, EdD, is the executive director of C-IMPACT.

Holly C. Wilcox, PhD, is a professor at the Johns Hopkins Bloomberg School of Public Health, the Johns Hopkins School of Medicine, and the Johns Hopkins School of Education.

References

Acosta, Joie, Matthew Chinman, Patricia Ebener, Patrick S. Malone, Andrea Phillips, and Asa Wilks. 2019. "Evaluation of a Whole-School Change Intervention: Findings from a Two-Year Cluster Randomized Trial of the Restorative Practices' Intervention." *Journal of Youth and Adolescence* 48 (5): 876–90. https://doi.org/10.1007/s10964-019-01013-2.

Addington, Lynn. 2014. "Surveillance and Security Approaches across School Levels." In *Responding to School Violence: Confronting the Columbine Effect*, edited by G. Muschert, G. Stuart Henry, N. L. Bracy, and A. A. Peguero, 71–88. Boulder, CO: Lynne Rienner.

Administration for Children and Families (ACF). 2019. *Head Start Program Facts: Fiscal Year 2019.* US Department of Health and Human Services, Office of Head Start.

Administration for Children and Families (ACF). 2020. *Preschool Development Grant Birth through Five Synthesis Report.* US Department of Health and Human Services, Office of Early Childhood Development.

Advocates for Children. 2015. *Civil Rights Suspended: An Analysis of New York City Charter School Discipline Policies.* New York: Advocates for Children. https://advocatesforchildren.org/wp-content/uploads/2024/03/civil_rights_suspended.pdf.

Agnich, Laura E. 2015. "A Comparative Analysis of Attempted and Completed School-Based Mass Murder Attacks." *American Journal of Criminal Justice: AJCJ* 40: 1–22. https://doi.org/10.1007/s12103-014-9239-5.

Ahmed, Shireen. 2018. "The Cutting of a Teenage Wrestler's Hair Was a Familiar Act of Violence for Black Athletes." *Guardian*, December 23, 2018. https://www.theguardian.com/sport/2018/dec/23/andrew-johnson-high-school-wrestler-dreadlocks-cut.

Alexander, Michelle. 2010. *The New Jim Crow: Mass Incarceration in the Age of Colorblindness*. New York: New Press.

Alliance for Children and Youth of Waterloo Region. n.d. *Strength-Based Approaches: Improving the Lives of Our Children and Youth.*

Althusser, Louis. 1969. "Ideology and Ideological State Apparatuses (notes towards an Investigation)." In *Lenin and Philosophy and Other Essays*. https://www.marxists.org/reference/archive/althusser/1970/ideology.htm.

Alvarez, Adam. 2020. "Seeing Race in the Research on Youth Trauma and Education: A Critical Review." *Review of Educational Research* 90, (5): 583–626.

Alvis, Monika. 2015. "Teachers' Perceptions about Using Restorative Practice-Based Programs in Schools." *Counselor Education Capstone* 4: 1–31.

American Academy of Pediatrics (AAP). 2021. "COVID-19 Guidance for Safe Schools and Promotion of In-Person Learning." https://www.aap.org/en/pages/2019-novel-coronavirus-covid-19-infections/clinical-guidance/covid-19-planning-considerations-return-to-in-person-education-in-schools/.

American Foundation for Suicide Prevention (AFSP). 2020. "State Laws: Suicide Prevention in Schools K–12." www.afsp.org.

American Foundation for Suicide Prevention, American School Counselor Association, National Association of School Psychologists and The Trevor Project. 2019. *Model School District Policy on Suicide Prevention: Model Language, Commentary, and Resources* (2nd ed.). New York: American Foundation for Suicide Prevention.

American Psychological Association (APA). 2018. "Racial Stress and Self-Care. Parent Tip Tool." RESilience Initiative. Retrieved from https://www.apa.org/res/parent-resources/racial-stress-tool-kit.pdf.

American Psychological Association Zero Tolerance Task Force. 2008. "Are Zero Tolerance Policies Effective in the Schools? An Evidentiary Review and Recommendations." *American Psychologist* 63 (9): 852–62. https://doi.org/10.1037/0003-066X.63.9.852.

Anderson, Kaitlin. 2018. "The Politics of School Discipline: A Quantitative

Analysis of the Legalization and Use of Corporal Punishment in the United States." *Journal of Public Management & Social Policy* 24 (2): 6.

Anderson, Kenneth Alonzo. 2018. "Does More Policing Make Middle Schools Safer?" *Brookings*. November 8, 2018. https://www.brookings.edu/articles/does-more-policing-make-middle-schools-safer/.

Anderson, Riana, Shawn Jones, Crystal Navarro, Monique McKenny, Tulsi Mehta, and Howard Stevenson. 2018. "Addressing the Mental Health Needs of Black American Youth and Families: A Case Study from the EMBRace Intervention." *International Journal of Environmental Research and Public Health* 15 (5): 898.

Anderson, Sara, Tama Leventhal, and Véronique Dupéré. 2014. "Exposure to Neighborhood Affluence and Poverty in Childhood and Adolescence and Academic Achievement and Behavior." *Applied Developmental Science* 18 (3): 123–38. https://doi.org/10.1080/10888691.2014.924355.

Annamma, Subini Ancy, Yolanda Anyon, Nicole M. Joseph, Jordan Farrar, Eldridge Greer, Barbara Downing, and John Simmons. 2019. "Black Girls and School Discipline: The Complexities of Being Overrepresented and Understudied." *Urban Education* 54 (2): 211–42.

Annie E. Casey Foundation. 2020. *Kids, Families and COVID-19: Pandemic Pain Points and the Urgent Need to Respond*. https://assets.aecf.org/m/resourcedoc/aecf-kidsfamiliesandcovid19-2020.pdf.

Antonio Aguirre, Bani, Mary Louise Z. Collins, and Megan E. Collins. 2021. "Vision Screening Requirements for School-Age Children during the COVID-19 Pandemic." *Ophthalmic Epidemiology* 29(6): 707–9. https://doi.org/10.1080/09286586.2021.2018714.

Anyon, Yolanda, Anne Gregory, Susan Stone, Jordan Farrar, Jeffrey M. Jenson, Jeanette McQueen, Barbara Downing, Eldridge Greer, and John Simmons. 2016. "Restorative Interventions and School Discipline Sanctions in a Large Urban School District." *American Educational Research Journal* 53(6): 1663–97. https://doi.org/10.3102/0002831216675719.

Armour, M. 2012. *Ed White Middle School Restorative Discipline Evaluation: Implementation and Impact, 2013/2014 Sixth & Seventh Grade*. The University of Texas at Austin. https://sites.utexas.edu/irjrd/files/2016/01/Year-2-Final-EW-Report.pdf.

Ascione, Laura. 2019. "Is Facial Recognition in Schools Reassuring—or Invasive?" *eSchool News*. February 28, 2019. https://www.eschoolnews.com/2019/02/28/facial-recognition-in-schools/.

Augustine, Catherine H., John Engberg, Geoffrey E. Grimm, Emma Lee, Elaine Lin Wang, Karen Christianson, and Andrea A. Joseph. 2018. *Can Restorative Practices Improve School Climate and Curb Suspensions? An Evaluation of the Impact of Restorative Practices in a Mid-Sized Urban School District*. RAND Corporation. https://www.rand.org/content/dam/rand/pubs/research_reports/RR2800/RR2840/RAND_RR2840.pdf.

Azevedo, Joao Pedro. 2020. "Learning Poverty in the Time of COVID-19." World Bank Group. https://openknowledge.worldbank.org/handle/10986/34850.

Bailey, Rebecca, Emily A. Meland, Gretchen Brion-Meisels, and Stephanie M. Jones. 2019. "Getting Developmental Science Back into Schools: Can What We Know about Self-Regulation Help Change How We Think about 'No Excuses'?" *Frontiers in Psychology* 10 (August): 1885. https://doi.org/10.3389/fpsyg.2019.01885.

Baldridge, Bianca J. 2020. "Negotiating Anti-Black Racism in 'Liberal' Contexts: The Experiences of Black Youth Workers in Community-Based Educational Spaces." *Race Ethnicity and Education* 23 (6): 747–66. https://doi.org/10.1080/13613324.2020.1753682.

Balingit, Moriah, Donna St. George, and Valerie Strauss. 2021. "As the New School Year Looms, Debates Over Mask Mandates Stir Anger and Confusion." *Washington Post*, July 30, 2021. https://www.washingtonpost.com/education/2021/07/29/school-masks-coronavirus/.

Balingit, Moriah, and Kate Rabinowitz. 2021. "Home Schooling Exploded among Black, Asian, and Latino Students. But It Wasn't Just the Pandemic." *Washington Post*, July 27, 2021. https://www.washingtonpost.com/education/2021/07/27/pandemic-homeschool-black-asian-hispanic-families/.

Baltimore's Promise. 2018. "Gaining Traction after High School Graduation: Understanding the Post-Secondary Pathways for Baltimore's Youth." https://www.baltimorespromise.org/psp.

Baron, E. J., E. G. Goldstein, and C. T. Wallace. 2020. "Suffering in Silence: How COVID-19 School Closures Inhibit the Reporting of Child Maltreatment."

Journal of Public Economics 190: 104258. https://doi.org/10.1016/j.jpubeco.2020.104258.

Barrish, Harriet H., Muriel Saunders, and Montrose M. Wolf. 1969. "Good Behavior Game: Effects of Individual Contingencies for Group Consequences on Disruptive Behavior in a Classroom." *Journal of Applied Behavior Analysis* 2 (2): 119–24.

Basile K. C., H. B. Clayton, S. DeGue, et al. 2020. "Interpersonal Violence Victimization among High School Students—Youth Risk Behavior Survey, United States, 2019." *Morbidity and Mortality Weekly Report* 69 (1): 28–37. http://dx.doi.org/10.15585/mmwr.su6901a4.

Bauer, Lauren. 2020a. "About 14 Million Children in the US Are Not Getting Enough to Eat." https://www.hamiltonproject.org/blog/about_14_million_children_in_the_us_are_not_getting_enough_to_eat.

Bauer, Lauren. 2020b. "The COVID-19 Crisis Has Already Left Too Many Children Hungry in America." *The Hamilton Project*. https://www.hamiltonproject.org/blog/the_covid_19_crisis_has_already_left_too_many_children_hungry_in_america.

Becker, Howard. 1963. *The Outsiders: Studies in the Sociology of Deviance*. New York: Free Press.

Benson, Peter L., and Peter C. Scales. 2009. "Positive Youth Development and the Prevention of Youth Aggression and Violence." *International Journal of Developmental Science* 3 (3): 218–34. https://doi.org/10.3233/dev-2009-3302.

Bernard, Donte L., Casey D. Calhoun, Devin E. Banks, Colleen A. Halliday, Chanita Hughes-Halbert, and Carla K. Danielson. 2021. "Making the 'C-ACE' for a Culturally Informed Adverse Childhood Experiences Framework to Understand the Pervasive Mental Health Impact of Racism on Black Youth." *Journal of Child & Adolescent Trauma* 14 (2): 233–47.

Bernard, Donte L., Lori S. Hoggard, and Enrique W. Neblett. 2018. "Racial Discrimination, Racial Identity, and Impostor Phenomenon: A Profile Approach." *Cultural Diversity & Ethnic Minority Psychology* 24 (1): 51–61. https://doi.org/10.1037/cdp0000161.

Bernardy, S., and R. Schmid. 2018. "Ensuring Students Feel Safe at School." *ACSA Resource Hub* (blog). *ACSA Resource Hub*. August 17, 2018. https://content.acsa.org/ensuring-students-feel-safe-at-school/.

Biden, J. 2021, March 2. *Remarks by President Biden on the Administration's COVID-19 Vaccination Efforts* [Speech audio transcript]. The White House. https://www.whitehouse.gov/briefing-room/speeches-remarks/2021/03/02/remarks-by-president-biden-on-the-administrations-covid-19-vaccination-efforts/.

Black, Derek W., and David Sciarra. 2020. "Betsy DeVos Just Crossed Another Line. She's an Ongoing Danger to Teachers and Students." *USA Today*, July 22, 2020. https://www.usatoday.com/story/opinion/2020/07/22/covid-19-reopening-schools-betsy-devos-dangerous-demands-column/5473465002/.

Blitz, Lisa V., Elizabeth M. Anderson, and Monique Saastamoinen. 2016. "Assessing Perceptions of Culture and Trauma in an Elementary School: Informing a Model for Culturally Responsive Trauma-Informed Schools." *The Urban Review* 48 (4): 520–542.

Blum, Robert W. 2003. "Positive Youth Development: A Strategy for Improving Adolescent Health." In *Handbook of Applied Developmental Science: Promoting Positive Child, Adolescent, and Family Development through Research, Policies, and Programs* (vol. 2), edited by Richard M. Lerner, Francine Jacobs, and Donald Wertlieb, 237–52. Sage.

Bonnell, Chris, Elizabeth Allen, Emily Warren, Jennifer McGowan, Leonardo Bevilacqua, Farah Jamal, Rosa Legood, et al. 2018. "Effects of the Learning Together Intervention on Bullying and Aggression in English Secondary Schools (INCLUSIVE): A Cluster Randomized Controlled Trial." *Lancet* 392 (10163), 2452–64. https://doi.org/10.1016/S0140- 6736(18)31782-3.

Borowsky, Iris Wagman, Marjorie Ireland, and Michael D. Resnick. 2001. "Adolescent Suicide Attempts: Risks and Protectors." *Pediatrics* 107 (3), 485–93. https://doi.org/10.1542/peds.107.3.485.

Borowsky, Iris Wagman, Michael D. Resnick, Marjorie Ireland, and Robert W. Blum. 1999. "Suicide Attempts among American Indian and Alaska Native Youth: Risk and Protective Factors." *Archives of Pediatrics & Adolescent Medicine* 153 (6): 573–80. https://doi.org/10.1001/archpedi.153.6.573.

Boullier, M., and M. Blair. 2018. "Adverse Childhood Experiences." *Pediatrics and Child Health* 28 (3): 132–37.

Bourdieu, Pierre. 1977. "Cultural Reproduction and Social Reproduction." In

Power and Ideology in Education, edited by J. Karabel and A. H. Halsey, 487–511. New York: Oxford University Press.

Bowles, Samuel, and Herbert Gintis. 1976. *Schooling in Capitalist America: Educational Reform and the Contradictions of Economic Life*. Basic Books.

Boyden, Jo, and Gillian Mann. 2005. "Children's Risk, Resilience, and Coping in Extreme Situations." In *Handbook for Working with Children and Youth: Pathways to Resilience Across Cultures and Contexts*, edited by Michael Ungar, 26. Sage.

Bradshaw, C. P., J. H. Zmuda, S. G. Kellam, and N. S. Ialongo. 2009. "Longitudinal Impact of Two Universal Preventive Interventions in First Grade on Educational Outcomes in High School." *Journal of Educational Psychology* 101 (4), 926–37. https://doi.org/10.1037/a0016586.

Bramer, Cristi A., Lynsey M. Kimmins, Robert Swanson, Jeremy Kuo, Patricia Vranesich, Lisa A. Jacques-Carroll, and Angela K. Shen. 2020. "Decline in Child Vaccination Coverage during the COVID-19 Pandemic – Michigan Care Improvement Registry, May 2016–May 2020." *American Journal of Transplantation* 20 (7): 1930–31. https://doi.org/10.1111/ajt.16112.

Brauner, Cheryl Boydell, and Cheryll Bowers Stephens. 2006. "Estimating the Prevalence of Early Childhood Serious Emotional/behavioral Disorders: Challenges and Recommendations." *Public Health Reports* 121 (3): 303–10. https://doi.org/10.1177/003335490612100314.

Brennan, Lauretta M., Daniel S. Shaw, Thomas J. Dishion, and Melvin Wilson. 2012. "Longitudinal Predictors of School-Age Academic Achievement: Unique Contributions of Toddler-Age Aggression, Oppositionality, Inattention, and Hyperactivity." *Journal of Abnormal Child Psychology* 40 (8): 1289–1300. https://doi.org/10.1007/s10802-012-9639-2.

Brent, D. A., M. Baugher, J. Bridge, T. Chen, and L. Chiappetta. 1999. "Age- and Sex-Related Risk Factors for Adolescent Suicide." *Journal of the American Academy of Child & Adolescent Psychiatry* 38 (12), 1497–1505.

Bridge, J. A., L. M. Horowitz, C. A. Fontanella, A. H. Sheftall, J. Greenhouse, K. J. Kelleher, and J. V. Campo. 2018. "Age-Related Racial Disparity in Suicide Rates among US Youths from 2001 through 2015." *JAMA Pediatrics* 172 (7): 697–99. https://doi.org/10.1001/jamapediatrics.2018.0399.

Brown, Ben. 2018. "Evaluations of School Policing Programs in the USA." In *The Palgrave International Handbook of School Discipline, Surveillance, and Social Control*, edited by Jo Deakin, Emmeline Taylor, and Aaron Kupchik, 327–49. Cham: Springer International Publishing. https://doi.org/10.1007/978-3-319-71559-9_17.

Brown, Christopher Pierce, Beth Smith Feger, and Brian Nelson Mowry. 2018. *RIGOROUS DAP in the Early Years: From Theory to Practice*. Redleaf Press.

Brown, L. 2016. "Two Baltimores: The White L vs. the Black Butterfly." *Baltimore Sun*.

Brown, Lawrence T. 2021. *The Black Butterfly: The Harmful Politics of Race and Space in America*. Johns Hopkins University Press.

Bruner, Charles. 2017. "ACE, Place, Race, and Poverty: Building Hope for Children." *Academic Pediatrics* 17 (7S): S123–29. https://doi.org/10.1016/j.acap.2017.05.009.

Brunson, Rod K., and Jody Miller. 2006. "Gender, Race, and Urban Policing: The Experience of African American Youths." *Gender & Society* 20 (4): 531–52.

Bryan, J., J. M. Williams, and D. Griffin. 2020. "Fostering Educational Resilience and Opportunities in Urban Schools through Equity-Focused School–Family–Community Partnerships." *Professional School Counseling* 23 (1_part_2): 2156759X19899179. https://doi.org/10.1177/2156759X19899179.

Buolamwini, Joy, and Timnit Gebru. 2018. "Gender Shades: Intersectional Accuracy Disparities in Commercial Gender Classification." *Proceedings of Machine Learning Research* 81, 1–15.

Burbio, Inc. 2021. K–12 School Opening Tracker. Retrieved March 25, 2022, from https://about.burbio.com/school-opening-tracker.

Burdick-Will, J., M. Keels, and T. Schuble. 2013. "Closing and Opening Schools: The Association between Neighborhood Characteristics and the Location of New Educational Opportunities in a Large Urban District." *Urban Affairs* 35 (1): 59–80.

Burke, Taylor A., Emily R. Kutok, Shira Dunsiger, Nicole R. Nugent, John V. Patena, Alison Riese, and Megan L. Ranney. 2021. "U.S. Adolescents' Mental Health and COVID-19-Related Changes in Technology Use, Fall 2020." medRxiv. https://doi.org/10.1101/2021.03.15.21253598.

Calear, A. L., and H. Christensen. 2010. "Systematic Review of School-Based Prevention and Early Intervention Programs for Depression." *Journal of Adolescents* 33, 429–38.

Cambria, N. 2011. "Deadly Day Cares Interactive: 45 Children Who Died." *St. Louis Post-Dispatch*, October 9, 2011. https://www.stltoday.com/news/special-reports/daycares/interactive-45-children-who-died/html_6b5ffd3e-85a5-11e0-93cd-0019bb30f31a.html.

Cameron, L., and M. Thorsborne. 2001. "Restorative Justice and School Discipline: Mutually Exclusive." *Restorative Justice and Civil Society* 180: 194.

Canady, Mo. 2018. "Standards and Best Practices for School Resource Officer Programs." National Association of School Resource Officers. https://www.nasro.org/clientuploads/About-Mission/NASRO-Standards-and-Best-Practices.pdf.

Cannon, J. S., M. R. Kilburn, L. A. Karoly, T. Mattox, A. N. Muchow, and M. Buenaventura. 2018. "Investing Early: Taking Stock of Outcomes and Economic Returns from Early Childhood Programs." *Rand Health Quarterly* 7 (4): 6.

Carli, Vladimir, Camilla Wasserman, Danuta Wasserman, Marco Sarchiapone, Alan Apter, Judit Balazs, Julio Bobes, et al. 2013. "The Saving and Empowering Young Lives in Europe (SEYLE) Randomized Controlled Trial (RCT): Methodological Issues and Participant Characteristics." *BMC Public Health* 13 (May): 479. https://doi.org/10.1186/1471-2458-13-479.

Carter, Prudence L., and Kevin G. Welner. 2013. *Closing the Opportunity Gap: What America Must Do to Give Every Child an Even Chance*. Oxford University Press.

Carter, Robert T., Veronica E. Johnson, Katheryn Roberson, Silvia L. Mazzula, Katherine Kirkinis, and Sinead Sant-Barket. 2017. "Race-Based Traumatic Stress, Racial Identity Statuses, and Psychological Functioning: An Exploratory Investigation." *Professional Psychology, Research and Practice* 48 (1): 30–37. https://doi.org/10.1037/pro0000116.

Cavanaugh, B. 2016. "Trauma-Informed Classrooms and Schools." *Beyond Behavior* 25 (2): 41–46.

Centers for Disease Control and Prevention (CDC). 2019. "Adverse Childhood Experiences (ACEs): Preventing Early Trauma to Improve Adult Health." *Vital Signs* 1–2.

Centers for Disease Control and Prevention (CDC). 2020a. *National Vital Statistics Reports* 69, no. 11. https://www.cdc.gov/nchs/data/nvsr/nvsr69/NVSR-69-11-508.pdf.

Centers for Disease Control and Prevention (CDC). 2020b. *Data & Statistics.* https://www.cdc.gov/healthyyouth/data/index.htm.

Centers for Disease Control and Prevention (CDC). 2021a. "CDC Releases 2019 Youth Risk Behavior Survey Results." August 2, 2021. https://www.cdc.gov/healthyyouth/data/yrbs/feature/index.htm.

Centers for Disease Control and Prevention (CDC). 2021b. "COVID Data Tracker" [data set]. https://covid.cdc.gov/covid-data-tracker/#cases_totalcases.

Centers for Disease Control and Prevention (CDC). 2021c. *Operational Strategy for K–12 Schools through Phased Prevention.* https://stacks.cdc.gov/view/cdc/106255.

Centers for Disease Control and Prevention (CDC). 2021d. *Provisional COVID-19 Deaths: Focus on Ages 0–18 Years* [data set]. National Center for Health Statistics. https://data.cdc.gov/NCHS/Provisional-COVID-19-Deaths-Focus-on-Ages-0-18-Yea/nr4s-juj3.

Centers for Disease Control and Prevention (CDC). 2021e. *Ventilation in Schools and Childcare Programs.* https://archive.cdc.gov/#/details?q=https://www.cdc.gov/coronavirus/2019-ncov/community/schools-childcare/ventilation.html&start=0&rows=10&url=https://www.cdc.gov/coronavirus/2019-ncov/community/schools-childcare/ventilation.html.

Centers for Disease Control and Prevention (CDC). 2021f. *Whole School, Whole Child, Whole Community (WSCC).* https: //www.cdc.gov/healthyschools/wscc/index.htm.

Centers for Disease Control and Prevention (CDC). 2022. "Disparities in Suicide." CDC. https://www.cdc.gov/suicide/disparities/?CDC_AAref_Val=https://www.cdc.gov/suicide/facts/disparities-in-suicide.html.

Centers for Disease Control and Prevention, National Center for Injury Prevention & Control. 2023. "WISQARS—Web-based Injury Statistics Query and Reporting System." www.cdc.gov/injury/wisqars.

Chafouleas, S. M., A. H. Johnson, S. Overstreet, and N. M. Santos. 2016. "Toward a Blueprint for Trauma-Informed Service Delivery in Schools." *School Mental Health* 8 (1): 144–62.

Chen, Grace. 2022. "Public School Police Departments: Combating Traffic, Crime and Budget Cuts." *Public School Review.* Updated May 18, 2022. https://www.publicschoolreview.com/blog/public-school-police-departments-combating-traffic-crime-and-budget-cuts.

Chetty, Raj, Nathaniel Hendren, Patrick Kline, Emmanuel Saez, and Nicholas Turner. 2014. "Is the United States Still a Land of Opportunity? Recent Trends in Intergenerational Mobility." *American Economic Review* 104 (5): 141–47. https://doi.org/10.1257/aer.104.5.141.

Children's Defense Fund. 1975. *School Suspensions: Are They Helping Children?* Cambridge, MA: Washington Research Project, Inc. https://files.eric.ed.gov/fulltext/ED113797.pdf.

Chinman, Matthew J., and Jean Ann Linney. 1998. "Toward a Model of Adolescent Empowerment: Theoretical and Empirical Evidence." *Journal of Primary Prevention* 18 (4): 393–413. https://doi.org/10.1023/A:1022691808354.

Chrusciel, Margaret, Scott E. Wolfe, J. Andrew Hansen, Robert J. Kaminski, and Jeff Rojek. 2015. "Law Enforcement Executive and Principal Perspectives on School Safety Measures: School Resource Officers and Armed School Employees." *Policing: An International Journal of Police Strategies & Management* 38 (1): 24–39.

Clark, Latoya Baldwin. 2022. "Barbed Wire Fences: The Structural Violence of Education Law." *The University of Chicago Law Review. University of Chicago. Law School* 89 (2): 499–524. https://chicagounbound.uchicago.edu/uclrev/vol89/iss2/8/.

Clark, Steven. 2011. "The Role of Law Enforcement in Schools: The Virginia Experience—a Practitioner Report." *New Directions for Youth Development* 2011 (129): 89–101. https://doi.org/10.1002/yd.389.

Clear, T. 2007. *Imprisoning Communities: How Mass Incarceration Makes Disadvantaged Neighborhoods Worse.* Oxford University Press.

Cohodes, Sarah. 2018. "Charter Schools and the Achievement Gap." *The Future of Children.* Princeton University and Brookings Institute, 1000 (1): 1–16. https://futureofchildren.princeton.edu/sites/g/files/toruqf2411/files/resource-links/charter_schools_compiled.pdf.

Coleman, J. S., E. Q. Campbell, C. J. Hobson, J. McPartland, A. M. Mood, F. D. Weinfeld, and R. L. York. 1966. "Equality of Educational Opportunity."

National Center for Educational Statistics, Office of Education, US Department of Health, Education and Welfare.

Committee for Economic Development (CED). 2019. *Child Care in State Economies*. Arlington, VA: CED.

Congress.gov. "H.R.1429 - 110th Congress (2007–2008): Improving Head Start for School Readiness Act of 2007." December 12, 2007. https://www.congress.gov/bill/110th-congress/house-bill/1429.

Congressional Black Caucus: Emergency Taskforce on Suicide. 2019. The McSilver Institute for Poverty Policy and Research at New York University. https://mcsilver.nyu.edu/taskforce-suicide/.

Connery, Chelsea. 2020. "The Prevalence and the Price of Police in Schools." Center for Education Policy Analysis, University of Connecticut. 2020. https://education.uconn.edu/2020/10/27/the-prevalence-and-the-price-of-police-in-schools/.

Corley, Cheryl. 2018. "Do Police Officers in Schools Really Make Them Safer?" *NPR*, March 8, 2018. https://www.npr.org/2018/03/08/591753884/do-police-officers-in-schools-really-make-them-safer.

Corrin, W., S. Sepanik, A. Gray, F. Fernandez, A. Briggs, and K. K. Wang. 2014. "Laying Tracks to Graduation: The First Year of Implementing Diplomas Now." *MDRC*. //efaidnbmnnnibpcajpcglclefindmkaj/https://mdrc.org/sites/default/files/Diplomas_Now_First_Year_FR_0.pdf.

Council on School Health, Jeffrey H. Lamont, Cynthia D. Devore, Mandy Allison, Richard Ancona, Stephen E. Barnett, Robert Gunther, Breena Holmes, Jeffrey H. Lamont, Mark Minier, Jeffrey K. Okamoto, Lani S. M. Wheeler, and Thomas Young. 2013. "Out-of-School Suspension and Expulsion." *Pediatrics*131 (3): e1000–e1007. https://doi.org/10.1542/peds.2012-3932.

Counts, Jennifer, Kristina N. Randall, Joseph B. Ryan, and Antonis Katsiyannis. 2018. "School Resource Officers in Public Schools: A National Review." *Education and Treatment of Children* 41, no. 4 (2018): 405–30. https://doi.org/10.1353/etc.2018.0023.

Craig, Shelley L. 2013. "Affirmative Supportive Safe and Empowering Talk (ASSET): Leveraging the Strengths and Resiliencies of Sexual Minority Youth in School-Based Groups." *Journal of LGBT Issues in Counseling* 7 (4): 372–86.

Craig, Shelley L., Ashley Austin, Jill Levenson, Vivian W. Leung, Andrew D. Eaton, and Sandra A. D'Souza. 2020. "Frequencies and Patterns of Adverse Childhood Events in LGBTQ Youth." *Child Abuse & Neglect* 107.

Crane M. A., R. R. Faden, and M. E. Collins. 2021. "How Are Teachers Prioritized for COVID-19 Vaccination by the US States?" *Johns Hopkins Berman Institute of Bioethics.* https://bioethics.jhu.edu/news-events/news/how-are-teachers-prioritized-for-covid-19-vaccination-by-the-us-states/.

Crouse, G., R. Ghertner, and N. Chien. 2023. "The Impact of the COVID-19 Pandemic on the Child Care Industry and Workforce." Office of Human Services Policy Brief. January 2023. Washington, DC. https://aspe.hhs.gov/sites/default/files/documents/71981d3ec3a1d02537d86d827806834b/Child-Care-Trends-COVID.pdf.

Cruz, R. A., and J. E. Rodl. 2018. "Crime and Punishment: An Examination of School Context and Student Characteristics That Predict Out-of-school Suspension." *Children and Youth Services Review* 95, 226–34.

Cuellar, Alison Evans, and Sara Markowitz. 2015. "School Suspension and the School-to-Prison Pipeline." *International Review of Law and Economics* 43 (August): 98–106. https://doi.org/10.1016/j.irle.2015.06.001.

Curran, F. Chris. 2016. "Estimating the Effect of State Zero Tolerance Laws on Exclusionary Discipline, Racial Discipline Gaps, and Student Behavior." *Educational Evaluation and Policy Analysis* 38 (4): 647–68. https://doi.org/10.3102/0162373716652728.

Curran, F. Chris, Benjamin W. Fisher, Samantha Viano, and Aaron Kupchik. 2019. "Why and When Do School Resource Officers Engage in School Discipline? The Role of Context in Shaping Disciplinary Involvement." *American Journal of Education* 126 (1): 33–63. https://doi.org/10.1086/705499.

Czyz, Ewa K., Zhuqing Liu, and Cheryl A. King. 2012. "Social Connectedness and One-Year Trajectories among Suicidal Adolescents Following Psychiatric Hospitalization." *Journal of Clinical Child & Adolescent Psychology* 41 (2): 214–26. https://doi.org/10.1080/15374416.2012.651998.

Daniels, Jeffrey A. 2019. "A Preliminary Report on the Police Foundations Averted School Violence Database." National Police Foundation.

Daniels, Jeffrey A., Karianne D. P. Bilksy, Susan Chamberlain, and Jennifer Haist. 2011. "School Barricaded Captive-Takings: An Exploratory Investigation of School Resource Officer Responses." *Psychological Services* 8 (3): 178–88. https://doi.org/10.1037/a0024738.

Darling-Hammond, S., T. A. Fronius, H. Sutherland, S. Guckenburg, A. Petrosino, and N. Hurley. 2020. "Effectiveness of Restorative Justice in US K–12 Schools: A Review of Quantitative Research." *Contemporary School Psychology* 24, 295–308.

Decker, Stacey. 2021. "Which States Banned Mask Mandates in Schools, and Which Required Masks?" *Education Week*, August 20, 2021. https://www.edweek.org/policy-politics/which-states-ban-mask-mandates-in-schools-and-which-require-masks/2021/08.

Dervic, K., D. A. Brent, and M. A. Oquendo. 2008. "Completed Suicide in Childhood." *Psychiatric Clinics of North America* 31 (2): 271–91. https://doi.org/10.1016/j.psc.2008.01.006.

Devlin, Deanna N., Mateus Rennó Santos, and Denise C. Gottfredson. 2018. "An Evaluation of Police Officers in Schools as a Bullying Intervention." *Evaluation and Program Planning* 71 (December): 12–21. https://doi.org/10.1016/j.evalprogplan.2018.07.004.

Dianis, Judith Browne. 2021. "The Police-Free Schools Movement Made Headway. Has It Lost Momentum?" *Education Week*, June 21, 2021. https://www.edweek.org/leadership/opinion-the-police-free-schools-movement-made-headway-has-it-lost-momentum/2021/06.

Diliberti, Melissa, Michael Jackson, Samuel Correa, and Zoe Padgett. 2019. "Crime, Violence, Discipline, and Safety in US Public Schools: Findings from the School Survey on Crime and Safety: 2017–18. First Look." NCES 2019–061. National Center for Education Statistics, July. http://files.eric.ed.gov/fulltext/ED596638.pdf.

Ditton, J. R. 1979. *Controlology: Beyond the New Criminology*. Springer.

Dodge, Kenneth A., Karen L. Bierman, John D. Coie, Mark T. Greenberg, John E. Lochman, Robert J. McMahon, and Ellen E. Pinderhughes. "Impact of Early Intervention on Psychopathology, Crime, and Well-Being at Age 25." *American Journal of Psychiatry* 172 (1): 59–70. https://doi.org/10.1176/appi.ajp.2014.13060786.

Doll, B., and M. A. Lyon. 1998. "Risk and Resilience: Implications for the Delivery of Educational and Mental Health Services in Schools." *School Psychology Review* 27 (3): 348–63.

Dooling K. 2020. *Phased Allocation of COVID-19 Vaccines* [Meeting]. ACIP 2020 Meeting, Atlanta, GA. https://www.cdc.gov/vaccines/acip/meetings/downloads/slides-2020-12/slides-12-20/02-COVID-Dooling-508.pdf.

Dorado, J. S., M. Martinez, L. E. McArthur, and T. Liebovitz. 2016. "Healthy Environments and Response to Trauma in Schools (HEARTS): A School-Based, Multi-Level Comprehensive Prevention and Intervention Program for Creating Trauma-Informed, Safe and Supportive Schools." *School Mental Health* 8, 163–76.

Dorn, E., B. Hancock, J. Sarakatsannis, and E. Viruleg. 2020. *COVID-19 and Student Learning in the United States: The Hurt Could Last a Lifetime.* McKinsey & Company. https://www.mckinsey.com/industries/public-and-social-sector/our-insights/covid-19-and-student-learning-in-the-united-states-the-hurt-could-last-a-lifetime.

Dray, J., J. Bowman, E. Campbell, M. Freund, L. Wolfenden, R. K. Hodder, K. McElwaine, et al. 2017. "Systematic Review of Universal Resilience-Focused Interventions Targeting Child and Adolescent Mental Health in the School Setting." *Journal of the American Academy of Child & Adolescent Psychiatry* 56 (10): 813–24.

Dumas, Michael J. 2014. "'Losing an Arm': Schooling as a Site of Black Suffering." *Race Ethnicity and Education* 17 (1): 1–29. https://doi.org/10.1080/13613324.2013.850412.

Dumas, Michael J. 2016. "Shutting Ish Down: Black Lives Matter as a Challenge to the Field of Education." *Division B Newsletter: Black Lives Matter* (pp. 7–10). AERA.

Dumas, Michael J., and Kihana Miraya ross. 2016. "'Be Real Black for Me': Imagining BlackCrit in Education." *Urban Education* 51 (4): 415–42. https://doi.org/10.1177/0042085916628611.

Dunlap, G., and L. Fox. 2015. "The Pyramid Model: PBS in Early Childhood Programs and Its Relation to School-Wide PBS." *Pyramid Model Consortium.*

Durkheim, Émile, Paul Fauconnet, Everett K. Wilson, Herman Schnurer, and Everett K. Wilson. 1961. *Moral Education: A Study in the Theory and Applica-*

tion of the Sociology of Education, translated by Herman Schnurer. New York: Free Press of Glencoe.

Education Week. 2020a. "Map: Where Were Schools Required to Be Open for the 2020–21 School Year?" July 28, 2020. https://www.edweek.org/leadership/map-where-are-schools-closed/2020/07.

Education Week. 2020b. "The Coronavirus Spring: The Historic Closing of US Schools (A Timeline)." Editorial Projects in Education, Inc. https://www.edweek.org/leadership/the-coronavirus-spring-the-historic-closing-of-u-s-schools-a-timeline/2020/07.

Education Week. 2021. "Most Students Now Have Home Internet Access. But What About Ones Who Don't?" 2021 Editorial Projects in Education, Inc. https://www.edweek.org/technology/most-students-now-have-home-internet-access-but-what-about-the-ones-who-dont/2021/04.

Egger, Helen Link, and Adrian Angold. 2006. "Common Emotional and Behavioral Disorders in Preschool Children: Presentation, Nosology, and Epidemiology." *Journal of Child Psychology and Psychiatry, and Allied Disciplines* 47 (3–4): 313–37. https://doi.org/10.1111/j.1469-7610.2006.01618.x.

Eisenberg, D. T., and A. W. Smith. 2020. *Restorative Practices in Baltimore City Schools: Research Updates and Implementation Guide.* Open Society Institute–Baltimore. https://digitalcommons.law.umaryland.edu/cgi/viewcontent.cgi?article=1004&context=cdrum_fac_pubs.

Epstein, Rebecca, Jamilia Blake, and Thalia Gonzalez. 2017. "Girlhood Interrupted: The Erasure of Black Girls' Childhood." Center on Poverty and Inequality, Georgetown Law.

Esserman, Dean. 2018. "The School Shootings That Don't Happen." National Policing Institute. https://www.policinginstitute.org/onpolicing/the-school-shootings-that-dont-happen/.

Ewing, E. 2020. *Ghosts in the Schoolyard: Racism and School Closings on Chicago's South Side.* Chicago: University of Chicago Press.

Faden, R. R. 2020. "Coronavirus Could Result in School Closings in the US. We Must Make Sure These Closings Meet the Needs of Low-Income Children." *Baltimore Sun*. https://www.baltimoresun.com/opinion/op-ed/bs-ed-op-0228-corona-virus-school-closings-ethics-20200227-wpapu2w2xfaujgkqcf3v7t26tq-story.html.

Fagen, M. C., and B. R. Flay. 2009. "Sustaining a School-Based Prevention Program: Results from the Aban Aya Sustainability Project." *Health Education & Behavior* 36 (1): 9–23.

Fallis, D. S., and A. Brittain. 2014. "Children at Risk: Unregulated Day Care in Virginia." *Washington Post*, August 30, 2014. https://www.washingtonpost.com/sf/investigative/2014/08/30/in-virginia-thousands-of-day-care-providers-receive-no-oversight/.

Fasching-Varner, Kenneth J., Roland W. Mitchell, Lori L. Martin, and Karen P. Bennett-Haron. 2014. "Beyond the School-to-Prison Pipeline and Toward an Educational and Penal Realism." *Equity & Excellence in Education* 47 (4): 410–429.

Federal Bureau of Investigation (FBI). 2020. *Active Shooter Incidents in the United States in 2019.* US Department of Justice. https://www.fbi.gov/file-repository/active-shooter-incidents-in-the-us-2019-042820.pdf/view.

Felitti, Vincent J., Robert F. Anda, Dale Nordenberg, David F. Williamson, Alison M. Spitz, Valerie Edwards, Mary P. Koss, and James S. Marks. 2019. "REPRINT OF: Relationship of Childhood Abuse and Household Dysfunction to Many of the Leading Causes of Death in Adults: The Adverse Childhood Experiences (ACE) Study." *American Journal of Preventive Medicine* 56 (6): 774–86. https://doi.org/10.1016/j.amepre.2019.04.001.

Fenwick-Smith, A., E. E. Dahlberg, and S. C. Thompson. 2018. "Systematic Review of Resilience-Enhancing, Universal, Primary School-Based Mental Health Promotion Programs." *BMC Psychology* 6 (1): 1–17.

Fergus, S., and M. A. Zimmerman. 2005. "Adolescent Resilience: A Framework for Understanding Healthy Development in the Face of Risk." *Annual Review Public Health* 26: 399–419.

Ferguson, Ann Arnett. 2001. *Bad Boys: Public Schools in the Making of Black Masculinity.* Ann Arbor: University of Michigan Press.

Ferguson, K. M., K. Bender, S. J. Thompson, B. Xie, and D. Pollio. 2012. "Exploration of Arrest Activity among Homeless Young Adults in Four US Cities." *Social Work Research* 36 (3): 233–38.

Fergusson, D. M., L. J. Woodward, and L. J. Horwood. 2000. "Risk Factors and Life Processes Associated with the Onset of Suicidal Behavior During Adolescence and Early Adulthood." *Psychological Medicine* 30 (1): 23–39. https://doi.org/10.1017/s003329179900135x.

Ferren, M. 2021. "Remote Learning and School Reopenings: What Worked and What Didn't." Center for American Progress. https://www.americanprogress.org/issues/education-k-12/reports/2021/07/06/501221/remote-learning-school-reopenings-worked-didnt/.

Ferriss, Susan. 2015. "An Epidemic of Questionable Arrests by School Police Soul-Searching in San Bernardino County Over Campus Cops' Tactics and Attitudes." *Huffington Post.* http://www.huffingtonpost.com/entry/san-bernadino-arrests_us_5669b21ce4b009377b24119e.

Finn, P., and J. McDevitt. 2005. "National Assessment of School Resource Officer Programs. Final Project Report. Document Number 209273." INS Reporter/Immigration and Naturalization Service, US Department of Justice. https://eric.ed.gov/?id=ED486268.

Fischer, S., and T. Orlowski. 2020. "Child Care Licensing Study, United States, 2017." *Inter-university Consortium for Political and Social Research*, 2020-09–08. https://doi.org/10.3886/ICPSR37700.v2.

Fisher, Benjamin W., and Emily A. Hennessy. 2016. "School Resource Officers and Exclusionary Discipline in U.S. High Schools: A Systematic Review and Meta-Analysis." *Adolescent Research Review* 1 (3): 217–33. https://doi.org/10.1007/s40894-015-0006-8.

Flanagan, Constance A., Amy K. Syvertsen, and Michael D. Stout. 2007. "Civic Measurement Models: Tapping Adolescents' Civic Engagement. CIRCLE Working Paper 55." *Center for Information and Research on Civic Learning and Engagement (CIRCLE)*, May. http://files.eric.ed.gov/fulltext/ED497602.pdf.

Fondren, K., M. Lawson, R. Speidel, C. G. McDonnell, and K. Valentino, K. 2020. "Buffering the Effects of Childhood Trauma Within the School Setting: A Systematic Review of Trauma-Informed and Trauma-Responsive Interventions Among Trauma-Affected Youth." *Children and Youth Services Review* 109 (February): 104691.

Fortson, Beverly L., National Center for Injury Prevention and Control (US) Division of Violence Prevention, Joanne Klevens, Melissa T. Merrick, Leah K. Gilbert, and Sandra P. Alexander. 2016. "Preventing Child Abuse and Neglect: A Technical Package for Policy, Norm, and Programmatic Activities." Centers for Disease Control and Prevention. https://doi.org/10.15620/cdc.38864.

Foucault, Michel. 1975. *Discipline and Punish. The Birth of the Prison*. New York: Vintage Books.

Fox, A. M., J. S. Lee, L. C. Sorensen, and E. G. Martin. 2021. "Sociodemographic Characteristics and Inequities Associated with Access to In-Person and Remote Elementary Schooling During the COVID-19 Pandemic in New York State." *JAMA Network Open* 4 (7): e2117267. https://doi.org/10.1001/jamanetworkopen.2021.17267.

Fox, Madeline, Kavitha Mediratta, Jessica Ruglis, Brett Stoudt, Seema Shah, and Michelle Fine. 2010. "Critical Youth Engagement: Participatory Action Research and Organizing." In *Handbook of Research on Civic Engagement in Youth*, edited by Lonnie R. Sherrod, Judith Torney-Purta, and Constance A. Flanagan, 621–49. Hoboken, NJ: John Wiley & Sons. https://doi.org/10.1002/9780470767603.ch23.

Frederique, Nadine. 2020. "What Do the Data Reveal about Violence in Schools?" National Institute of Justice. https://nij.ojp.gov/topics/articles/what-do-data-reveal-about-violence-schools.

Friedman-Krauss, A. H., S. Barnett, K. A. Garver, K. S. Hodges, G. G. Weisenfeld, and B. A. Gardiner. 2020. "The State of Preschool 2019: State Preschool Yearbook." National Institute for Early Education Research. https://irp-cdn.multiscreensite.com/5877256e/files/uploaded/YB2019_Full_Report.pdf.

García, J. L., J. J. Heckman, D. E. Leaf, and M. J. Prados. 2016. *The Life-Cycle Benefits of an Influential Early Childhood Program*. NBER Working Paper No. 22993, JEL No. C93, I28, J13.

Garcia-Area, Patricia, and Stephanie D'Souza, S. 2020. "Spotlight on English Learners." *American Institutes for Research*. https://www.air.org/sites/default/files/COVID-Survey-Spotlight-on-English-Learners-FINAL-Oct-2020.pdf

Garnett, Bernice, Mika Moore, Jon Kidde, Tracy A. Ballysingh, Colby T. Kervick, Lisa Bedinger, Lance C. Smith, and Henri Sparks. 2020. "Needs and Readiness Assessments for Implementing School-Wide Restorative Practices." *Improving Schools* 23 (1): 21–32. https://doi.org/10.1177/1365480219836529.

Garofalo, R., R. C. Wolf, L. S. Wissow, E. R. Woods, and E. Goodman. 1999. "Sexual Orientation and Risk of Suicide Attempts among a Representative Sample of Youth." *Archives of Pediatrics and Adolescent Medicine* 153 (5): 487–93. https://doi.org/10.1001/archpedi.153.5.487.

Gayle, H., W. Foege, L. Brown, and B. Kahn. (Eds.). 2020. *Framework for Equitable Allocation of COVID-19 Vaccine.* National Academies of Sciences, Engineering, and Medicine, National Academies Press. https://doi.org/10.17226/25917.

Gay, Lesbian & Straight Education Network and Gay Straight Alliance Network (GLSEN). 2021. "New Research Shows Positive Impact of Gender and Sexuality Alliances in Schools." GLSEN. https://www.glsen.org/news/new-research-shows-positive-impact-gender-and-sexuality-alliances-schools.

Gay, Lesbian & Straight Education Network and Gay Straight Alliance Network (GLSEN). 2022. "GSA Resources." GLSEN. https://www.glsen.org/support-student-gsas.

Ghavami, Negin, Bryan E. Thornton, and Sandra Graham. 2021. "School Police Officers' Roles: The Influence of Social, Developmental and Historical Contexts." *Journal of Criminal Justice* 72: 101724. https://doi.org/10.1016/j.jcrimjus.2020.101724.

Gilbert, Leah K., Tara W. Strine, Leigh E. Szucs, Tamara N. Crawford, Sharyn E. Parks, Danielle T. Barradas, Rashid Njai, and Jean Y. Ko. 2020. "Racial and Ethnic Differences in Parental Attitudes and Concerns about School Reopening during the COVID-19 Pandemic – United States, July 2020." *Morbidity and Mortality Weekly Report* 69 (49): 1848–52. https://doi.org/10.15585/mmwr.mm6949a2.

Gilliam, Walter S., and Golan Shahar. 2006. "Preschool and Child Care Expulsion and Suspension." *Infants and Young Children*. https://doi.org/10.1097/00001163-200607000-00007.

Ginwright, S., and J. Cammarota. 2002. "New Terrain in Youth Development: The Promise of a Social Justice Approach." *Social Justice* 29 (4): 82–95. http://www.jstor.org/stable/29768150.

Gleason, Phillip, Melissa Clark, Christina C. Tuttle, Emily Dwoyer, and Marsha Silverberg. 2010. "The Evaluation of Charter School Impacts." *Institute of Education Sciences.* Washington, DC: US Department of Education. https://ies.ed.gov/ncee/pubs/20104029/pdf/20104030.pdf.

Golann, Joanne W. 2015. "The Paradox of Success at a No-Excuses School." *Sociology of Education* 88 (2): 103–19. https://doi.org/10.1177/0038040714567866.

Golann, Joanne W. 2021. "Opinion: Why Are No-Excuses Schools Moving

Beyond No Excuses? Charter Networks Like KIPP, Noble and Achievement First Rethink Strict Discipline." *The Hechinger Report*. https://hechinger report.org/opinion-why-are-no-excuses-schools-moving-beyond-no-excuses/.

Golann, Joanne, and Mira Debs. 2019. "The Harsh Discipline of No-Excuses Charter Schools: Is It Worth the Promise?" *Education Week*, June 9, 2019. https://www.edweek.org/leadership/opinion-the-harsh-discipline-of-no-excuses-charter-schools-is-it-worth-the-promise/2019/06.

Goldenberg, B. M. 2014. "White Teachers in Urban Classrooms: Embracing Non-White Students' Cultural Capital for Better Teaching and Learning." *Urban Education* 49 (1): 111–44.

Goldstein, Dana. 2020. "Do Police Officers Make Schools Safer or More Dangerous?" *New York Times*, June 12, 2020. https://www.nytimes.com/2020/06/12/us/schools-police-resource-officers.html.

Goldstein, N. E., L. M. Cole, M. Houck, E. Haney-Caron, S. Brooks-Holliday, R. Kreimera, and K. Bethel. 2019. "Dismantling the School to Prison Pipeline: The Philadelphia Police School Diversion Program." *Children and Youth Services Review* 101 (June), 61–69.

Gomez, B. J., and P. M. Ang. 2007. "Promoting Positive Youth Development in Schools." *Theory into Practice* 46 (2): 97–104.

Gonzalez, A., N. Monzon, D. Solis, L. Jaycox, and A. K. Langley. 2016. "Trauma Exposure in Elementary School Children: Description of Screening Procedures, Level of Exposure, and Posttraumatic Stress Symptoms." *School Mental Health* 8 (1): 77–88.

Goodenow, Carol, Laura Szalacha, and Kim Westheimer. 2006. "School Support Groups, Other School Factors, and the Safety of Sexual Minority Adolescents." *Psychology in the Schools* 43: 573–89. https://doi.org/10.1002/pits.20173.

González, T. 2015. "Socializing Schools: Addressing Racial Disparities in Discipline through Restorative Justice. In *Closing the School Discipline Gap: Equitable Remedies for Excessive Exclusion*, edited by D. Losen, 151–65. Teachers College Press.

González, T., H. Sattler, and A. J. Buth. 2019. "New Directions in Whole-School Restorative Justice Implementation." *Conflict Resolution Quarterly* 36 (3): 207–20.

Gottfredson, Denise C., Scott Crosse, Zhiqun Tang, Erin L. Bauer, Michele A. Harmon, Carol A. Hagen, and Angela D. Greene. 2020. "Effects of School Resource Officers on School Crime and Responses to School Crime." *Criminology and Public Policy* 19 (3): 905–40. https://doi.org/10.1111/1745-9133.12512.

Gould, E., and H. Blair. 2020. *Who's Paying Now? The Explicit and Implicit Costs of the Current Early Care and Education System*. Economic Policy Institute and Center for the Study of Child Care Employment, University of California Berkeley. https://www.epi.org/publication/whos-paying-now-costs-of-the-current-ece-system/.

Governor's Office of Crime Control and Prevention. 2019. *Maryland's Annual Disproportionate Minority Contact Plan FY 2019*.

Graham-Bermann, S. A., and H. M. Halabu. 2004. "Fostering Resilient Coping in Children Exposed to Violence: Cultural Considerations." In *Protecting Children from Domestic Violence: Strategies for Community Intervention*, edited by P. G. Jaffe, L. L. Baker, and A. J. Cunningham, 71–88. Guilford Press.

Gramsci, A. 1999. "Selections from Prison Notebooks." Retrieved on September 17, 2019, from http://courses.justice.eku.edu/pls330_louis/docs/gramsci-prison-notebooks-vol1.pdf.

Grant, A. A. 2020. "Testing the Promise of Restorative Practices for Reducing Teacher Turnover in Hard-to-Staff Schools." Unpublished doctoral dissertation, Johns Hopkins University, Baltimore, MD.

Grant, A. A., and D. J. Mac Iver. 2021. "Restorative Practices as a Social Justice Intervention in Urban Secondary Schools: Impacts and Challenges." In *Handbook of Social Justice Interventions in Education*, edited by C. A. Mullen, 741–62. Springer International Publishing.

Grant, Ashley A., Douglas J. Mac Iver, and Martha Abele Mac Iver. 2022. "The Impact of Restorative Practices with Diplomas Now on School Climate and Teachers' Turnover Intentions: Evidence from a Cluster Multi-Site Randomized Control Trial." *Journal of Research on Educational Effectiveness* 15 (3): 445–74. https://doi.org/10.1080/19345747.2021.2018745.

Grant, A. A., D. J. Mac Iver, V. Byrnes, E. Clark, R. Balfanz, and R. Lofton. 2023. "Combining Restorative Practices with Diplomas Now: Impacts on Schools' Practices, Problems, Suspensions, and Chronic Absenteeism." *Journal of*

Education for Students Placed at Risk. https://doi.org/10.1080/10824669.2023.2278047.

Greenberg, Sheldon F. 2017. *Frontline Policing in the 21st Century: Mastery of Police Patrol.* Springer, Palgrave Macmillan.

Gregory, A., K. Clawson, A. Davis, and J. Gerewitz. 2016. "The Promise of Restorative Practices to Transform Teacher-Student Relationships and Achieve Equity in School Discipline." *Journal of Educational and Psychological Consultation* 26 (4): 325–53.

Gregory, Ted. 2018. "Outcomes in School Shootings Can Differ Wildly Despite Presence of Resource Officers." *Chicago Tribune*, May 18, 2018. https://www.chicagotribune.com/news/ct-met-school-shootings-resource-officers-20180518-story.html.

Griffith, Janelle. 2020. "Black Texas Teen Told to Cut His Dreadlocks to Walk at Graduation." NBC News. January 23, 2020. https://www.nbcnews.com/news/us-news/black-texas-teen-told-cut-his-dreadlocks-order-walk-graduation-n1120731.

Grogger, J., and M. Willis. 2000. "The Emergence of Crack Cocaine and the Rise in Urban Crime Rates." *The Review of Economics and Statistics* 82 (4): 519–29.

Gross, Betheny, and Alice Opalka. 2020. "Too Many Schools Leave Learning to Chance during the Pandemic." Center for Reinventing Public Education. https://americanprogress.org/article/remote-learning-school-reopenings-worked-didnt/

Gupta, Sonia, and Manveen Kaur Jawanda. 2020. "The Impacts of COVID-19 on Children." *Acta Paediatrica* 109 (11): 2181–83. https://doi.org/10.1111/apa.15481.

Haider, A. 2021. "The Basic Facts About Children in Poverty." Center for American Progress. https://www.americanprogress.org/issues/poverty/reports/2021/01/12/494506/basic-facts-children-poverty/.

Harlem Lacrosse. 2020. "Harlem Lacrosse Annual Report." https://www.harlemlacrosse.org.

Harris, C. 1993. "Whiteness as Property." *Harvard Law Review* 106 (8): 1707–91. https://harvardlawreview.org/1993/06/whiteness-as-property/.

Hart, L. M., P. Cropper, A. J. Morgan, C. M. Kelly, and A. F. Jorm. 2020. "Teen Mental Health First Aid as a School-Based Intervention for Improving Peer

Support of Adolescents at Risk of Suicide: Outcomes from a Cluster Randomized Crossover Trial." *Australian and New Zealand Journal of Psychiatry* 54 (4): 382–92. https://doi.org/10.1177/0004867419885450.

Hart, L. M., A. J. Morgan, A. Rossetto, C. M. Kelly, A. Mackinnon, and A. F. Jorm. 2018. "Helping Adolescents to Better Support Their Peers with a Mental Health Problem: A Cluster-Randomized Crossover Trial of Teen Mental Health First Aid." *Australian and New Zealand Journal of Psychiatry* 52 (7): 638–51. https://doi.org/10.1177/0004867417753552.

Hartman, S. V. 1997. *Scenes of Subjection: Terror, Slavery, and Self-Making in Nineteenth-Century America.* Oxford University Press.

Harvey, David. 2007. *A Brief History of Neoliberalism.* Oxford University Press.

Hawton, K., K. E. Saunders, and R. C. O'Connor. 2012. "Self-Harm and Suicide in Adolescents." *Lancet* (London, England) 379 (9834): 2373–82. https://doi.org/10.1016/S0140-6736(12)60322-5.

Heck, N. C. 2015. "The Potential to Promote Resilience: Piloting a Minority Stress-Informed, GSA-Based, Mental Health Promotion Program for LGBTQ Youth." *Psychology of Sexual Orientation and Gender Diversity* 2 (3): 225.

Henderson, N., and M. M. Milstein. 2003. *Resiliency in Schools: Making It Happen for Students and Educators.* Corwin Press.

Henig, Jeffrey R. 2008. "What Do We Know about the Outcomes of KIPP Schools?" National Education Policy Center. http://nepc.colorado.edu/publication/outcomes-of-kipp-schools.

Henig, Jeffrey, Richard Hula, Marion Orr, and Desiree Pedescleaux. 2001. *The Color of School Reform: Race, Politics, and the Challenge of Urban Education.* Princeton, NJ: Princeton University Press.

Herring, Chris. 2019. "Concentrated Poverty." *The Wiley Blackwell Encyclopedia of Urban and Regional Studies,* 1–10. https://doi.org/10.1002/9781118568446.eurs0061.

Himmelstein, Kathryn E. W., and Hannah Brückner. 2011. "Criminal-Justice and School Sanctions against Nonheterosexual Youth: A National Longitudinal Study." *Pediatrics* 127 (1): 49–57. https://doi.org/10.1542/peds.2009-2306.

Hirschi, Travis. 2001. *Causes of Delinquency.* Somerset, NJ: Transaction.

Hobbs, Tawnell D. 2020. "Schools Are Reopening, Then Quickly Closing Due to

Coronavirus Outbreaks." *Wall Street Journal*, August 17, 2020. https://www.wsj.com/articles/schools-are-reopening-then-quickly-closing-due-to-coronavirus-outbreaks-11597700886.

Hodder, R. K., M. Freund, L. Wolfenden, J. Bowman, S. Nepal, J. Dray, M. Kingsland, et al. 2017. "Systematic Review of Universal School-Based 'Resilience' Interventions Targeting Adolescent Tobacco, Alcohol, or Illicit Substance Use: A Meta-Analysis." *Preventive Medicine* 100, 248–68.

Hoffmann, J. A., C. A. Farrell, M. C. Monuteaux, E. W. Fleegler, and L. K. Lee. 2020. "Association of Pediatric Suicide with County-Level Poverty in the United States, 2007–2016." *JAMA Pediatrics* 174 (3): 287–94. https://doi.org/10.1001/jamapediatrics.2019.5678.

Hough, Heather. 2021. "COVID-19, the Educational Equity Crisis, and the Opportunity Ahead." The Brookings Institution. https://www.brookings.edu/blog/brown-center-chalkboard/2021/04/29/covid-19-the-educational-equity-crisis-and-the-opportunity-ahead/.

Houry, D. E., and J. A. Mercy. 2019. "Preventing Adverse Childhood Experiences (ACEs): Leveraging the Best Available Evidence." Atlanta, GA: Centers for Disease Control and Prevention.

Hughes, K., M. A. Bellis, K. A. Hardcastle, D. Sethi, A. Butchart, C. Mikton, L. Jones, et al. 2017. "The Effect of Multiple Adverse Childhood Experiences on Health: A Systematic Review and Meta-Analysis." *The Lancet Public Health* 2 (8): e356–e366.

Hunt, Jerome, and Aisha C. Moodie-Mills. 2012. "The Unfair Criminalization of Gay and Transgender Youth: An Overview of the Experiences of LGBT Youth in the Juvenile Justice System." June 29, 2012. Center for American Progress

Hussar, B., J. Zhang, S. Hein, K. Wang, A. Roberts, J. Cui, M. Smith, F. Bullock Mann, A. Barmer, and R. Dilig. 2020. *The Condition of Education 2020* (NCES 2020-144). US Department of Education. Washington, DC: National Center for Education Statistics. https://nces.ed.gov/pubsearch/pubsinfo.asp?pubid=2020144.

Hutchinson, Asa. 2013. "Report of the National School Shield Task Force." National School Shield. https://www.edsource.org/wp-content/uploads/old/NSS_Final.pdf.

Ibrahim, Habiba, David L Barnes, Sheretta T. Butler-Barnes, and Odis Johnson Jr. 2021. "Impact of In-School Suspension on Black Girls' Math Course-Taking in High School." *Social Sciences* 10, 272. https://par.nsf.gov/servlets/purl/10316704.

Improving America's Schools Act of 1994, G. F. S. 1994. Public Law 103–382, 108 Statute 3907.

Institute of Medicine and National Research Council. 2015. "Government Investments in Marginalized Young Adults. National Academies Press (US)." https://www.ncbi.nlm.nih.gov/books/NBK284797/.

Institute on Trauma and Trauma-Informed Care. 2015. "What Is Trauma-Informed Care?" 2015. https://socialwork.buffalo.edu/social-research/institutes-centers/institute-on-trauma-and-trauma-informed-care/what-is-trauma-informed-care.html.

International Institute for Restorative Practices. 2011. *SaferSanerSchools: Whole-School Change through Restorative Practices.* https://www.iirp.edu/pdf/WSC-Overview.pdf.

International Institute for Restorative Practices. 2020. *IIRP Factbook: 2018–2019 Academic Year.* https://www.iirp.edu/images/pdf/IIRP_Factbook_AY-2018–19.pdf.

Irwin, V., K. Wang, J. Cui, J. Zhang, and A. Thompson. 2021. "Report on Indicators of School Crime and Safety: 2020 (NCES 2021–092/NCJ 300772)." National Center for Education Statistics, US Department of Education, and Bureau of Justice Statistics, Office of Justice Programs, US Department of Justice. Washington, DC. Retrieved August 1, 2021, from https://nces.ed.gov/pubsearch/pubsinfo.asp?pubid=2021092.

Jabbari, Jason, and Odis Johnson Jr. 2020. "The Collateral Damage of In-School Suspensions: A Counterfactual Analysis of High-Suspension Schools, Math Achievement and College Attendance." *Urban Education*, 0042085920902256. https://doi.org/10.1177/0042085920902256.

Jackson, D., and J. Bowdon. 2020. "Spotlight on Students with Disabilities." *American Institutes for Research.* https://www.air.org/sites/default/files/COVID-Survey-Spotlight-on-Students-with-Disabilities-FINAL-Oct-2020.pdf.

Jackson, M., M. Diliberti, J. Kemp, S. Hummel, C. Cox, K. Gbondo-Tugbawa,

D. Simon, and R. Hansen. 2018. *2015–16 School Survey on Crime and Safety (SSOCS): Public use data file user's manual (NCES 2018–107).* US Department of Education, National Center for Education Statistics. http://nces.ed.gov/pubsearch.

Jain, S., H. Bassey, M. Brown, and P. Kalra. 2014. *Restorative Justice in Oakland Schools: Implementation and Impacts.* Oakland Unified School District. https://www.nycourts.gov/ip/justiceforchildren/PDF/RestorativePracticeConf/P4-Davis-RJ_OUSD_Implementation.pdf.

James, Nathan, and Gail McCallion. 2013. "School Resource Officers: Law Enforcement Officers in Schools." Congressional Research Service.

Janowitz, M. 1975/1991. *On Social Organization and Social Control.* Chicago: University of Chicago Press.

Jargowsky, Paul. A. 2013. "Concentration of Poverty in the New Millennium: Changes in the Prevalence, Composition, and Location of High-Poverty Neighborhoods." The Century Foundation and Rutgers Center for Urban Research and Education.

Jencks, Christopher, and Susan E. Mayer. 1990. "The Social Consequences of Growing Up in a Poor Neighborhood." *Inner-City Poverty in the United States* 111: 186.

Jennings, Louise B., Deborah M. Parra-Medina, Deanne K. Hilfinger-Messias, and Kerry McLoughlin. 2006. "Toward a Critical Social Theory of Youth Empowerment." *Journal of Community Practice* 14 (1–2): 31–55. https://doi.org/10.1300/j125v14n01_03.

Jeon, L., E. Hur, K. Ardeleanu, T. Satchell, and C. R. Swanson. 2021. "Early Childhood Professionals' Psychological Well-Being." In *Contemporary Perspectives on Research on Child Care in Early Childhood Education*, edited by O. N. Saracho, 63–84. Charlotte, NC: Information Age Publishing.

Jessen-Howard, Steven, Rasheed Malik, and M. K. Falgout. 2020. "Costly and Unavailable: America Lacks Sufficient Childcare Supply for Infants and Toddlers." Center for American Progress. Washington: DC. https://www.americanprogress.org/issues/early-childhood/reports/2020/08/04/488642/costly-unavailable-america-lacks-sufficient-child-care-supply-infants-toddlers/.

Jimenez, Manuel E., Roy Wade Jr., Yong Lin, Lesley M. Morrow, and Nancy E.

Reichman. 2016. "Adverse Experiences in Early Childhood and Kindergarten Outcomes." *Pediatrics* 137 (2): e20151839. https://doi.org/10.1542/peds.2015-1839.

Johns, M. M., R. Lowry, L. T. Haderxhanaj, C. N. Rasberry, L. Robin, L. Scales, D. Stone, and N. A. Suarez. 2020. "Trends in Violence Victimization and Suicide Risk by Sexual Identity Among High School Students – Youth Risk Behavior Survey, United States, 2015–2019." *Morbidity and Mortality Weekly Report* 69 (1): 19–27. https://doi.org/10.15585/mmwr.su6901a3.

Johnson, Odis Jr. 2015. "Responding to School Violence: Confronting the Columbine Effect." *Contemporary Sociology* 44 (4): 539–41.

Johnson, Odis Jr., and Jason Jabbari. 2021. "The Infrastructure of Black Social Control: A Multi-Level Counterfactual Analysis of Surveillance, Punishment, and Educational Inequality." AERA Conference Paper.

Johnson, Odis Jr., and Jason Jabbari. 2022. "The Racialized Interaction of School Suspension, Math Performance, and Math Self-Efficacy in Majority White Schools." *Educational Forum*.

Johnson, Odis, Jason Jabbari, Maya Williams, and Olivia Marcucci. 2019. "Disparate Impacts: Balancing the Need for Safe Schools with Racial Equity in Discipline." *Policy Insights from the Behavioral and Brain Sciences* 6 (2): 162–69. https://doi.org/10.1177/2372732219864707.

Jones, Damon E., Mark Greenberg, and Max Crowley. 2015. "Early Social-Emotional Functioning and Public Health: The Relationship Between Kindergarten Social Competence and Future Wellness." *American Journal of Public Health* 105 (11): 2283–90. https://doi.org/10.2105/AJPH.2015.302630.

Joseph, George, and CityLab. 2016. "Charter Schools in Black Areas Suspend More Often." *The Atlantic*, September 16, 2016. https://www.theatlantic.com/education/archive/2016/09/the-racism-of-charter-school-discipline/500240/.

Karp, D. R., and B. Breslin. 2001. "Restorative Justice in School Communities." *Youth and Society* 33 (2): 249–72.

Kataoka, S., L. H. Jaycox, M. Wong, E. Nadeem, A. Langley, L. Tang, and B. D. Stein. 2011. "Effects on School Outcomes in Low-Income Minority Youth: Preliminary Findings from a Community-Partnered Study of a School-Based

Trauma Intervention." *Ethnicity and Disease* 21 (3 Suppl 1), S1–S71–7. https://www.ncbi.nlm.nih.gov/pubmed/22352083.

Kellam, S. G., C. H. Brown, J. M. Poduska, N. S. Ialongo, W. Wang, P. Toyinbo, et al. 2008. "Effects of a Universal Classroom Behavior Management Program in First and Second Grades on Young Adult Behavioral, Psychiatric, and Social Outcomes." *Drug and Alcohol Dependence* 95: S5–S28.

Kellam, S. G., X. Ling, R. Merisca, C. H. Brown, and N. Ialongo. 1998. "The Effect of the Level of Aggression in the First-Grade Classroom on the Course and Malleability of Aggressive Behavior into Middle School." *Development and Psychopathology* 10: 165–85.

Kellam, S. G., Rebok, G. W., Wilson, R., Mayer, L. S. 1994. "The Social Field of the Classroom: Context for the Developmental Epidemiological Study of Aggressive Behavior." In *Adolescence in Context: The Interplay of Family, School, Peers, and Work in Adjustment*, edited by R. K. Silbereisen and E. Todt, 390–408. New York: Springer-Verlag.

Kerstetter, K. 2016. "A Different Kind of Discipline: Social Reproduction and the Transmission of Non-Cognitive Skills at an Urban Charter School." *Sociological Inquiry* 86 (4): 512–39.

Keyes, K. M., A. Hamilton, M. E. Patrick, and J. Schulenberg. 2020. "Diverging Trends in the Relationship between Binge Drinking and Depressive Symptoms Among Adolescents in the U.S. from 1991 through 2018." *Journal of Adolescent Health* 66 (5): 529–35. https://doi.org/10.1016/j.jadohealth.2019.08.026.

Kids Count Data Center. 2020. *Children in Poverty (100 percent poverty) in the United States* [data set]. Annie. E. Casey Foundation. https://datacenter.kidscount.org/data/tables/43-children-in-poverty-100-percent-poverty#detailed/1/any/false/1729,37,871,870,573,869,36,868,867,133/any/321,322.

Kim, Catherine Y., Daniel J. Losen, and Damon T. Hewitt. 2010. *The School-to-Prison Pipeline: Structuring Legal Reform*. NYU Press.

Kim, Lindsay, Michael Whitaker, Alissa O'Halloran, et al. 2020. "Hospitalization Rates and Characteristics of Children Aged < 18 Years Hospitalized with Laboratory-Confirmed COVID-19—COVID-NET, 14 States, March 1–July 25, 2020." *Morbidity and Mortality Weekly Report* 69 (32): 1081. https://doi.org/10.15585/mmwr.mm6932e3.

Kirk, David S. 2009. "Unraveling the Contextual Effects on Student Suspension and Juvenile Arrest: The Independent and Interdependent Influences of School, Neighborhood, and Family Social Controls." *Criminology: An Interdisciplinary Journal* 47 (2): 479–520. https://doi.org/10.1111/j.1745-9125.2009.00147.x.

Kleinman, R. E., J. M. Murphy, M. Little, M. Pagano, C. A. Wehler, K. Regal, and M. S. Jellinek. 1998. "Hunger in Children in the United States: Potential Behavioral and Emotional Correlates." *Pediatrics* 101 (1): E3. http://pediatrics.aappublications.org/content/101/1/e3.long.

Korman, H. T., B. O'Keefe, and M. Repka. 2020. *Missing in the Margins: Estimating the Scale of the COVID-19 Attendance Crisis.* Bellwether Education Partners.

Kranz, A. M., E. D. Steiner, and J. M. Mitchell. 2022. "School-Based Health Services in Virginia and the COVID-19 Pandemic." *Journal of School Health* 92 (5): 436–44. https://doi.org/10.1111/josh.13147.

Kress, Cathann. 2004. "The Essential Elements of 4-H Youth Development." 4-H. https://4-h.org/wp-content/uploads/2016/02/WindPDFs-EssentialsNEW.pdf.

Kuhfeld, Megan, Jim Soland, Beth Tarasawa, Angela Johnson, Erik Ruzek, and Karyn Lewis. 2020. "How Is COVID-19 Affecting Student Learning: Initial Findings from Fall 2020." The Brookings Institution. https://www.brookings.edu/blog/brown-center-chalkboard/2020/12/03/how-is-covid-19-affecting-student-learning/.

Kumi-Yeboah, A., A. C. Onyewuenyi, and P. Smith. 2021. "Teaching Black Immigrant Students in Urban Schools: Teacher and Peer Relationships and Academic Performances." *Urban Review* 53 (2): 218–42.

Kupchik, Aaron. 2020. "Counselors and Mental-Health Workers Can Make a Bigger Difference Than SROs." *Delaware News Journal*, June 27, 2020. https://www.delawareonline.com/story/opinion/2020/06/27/counselors-and-mental-healthworkers-can-make-bigger-difference/3258330001.

Lacombe, Dany. 1996. "Reforming Foucault: A Critique of the Social Control Thesis." *The British Journal of Sociology* 47 (2): 332–52. https://doi.org/10.2307/591730.

Ladson-Billings, G. 2006. "From the Achievement Gap to the Education Debt:

Understanding Achievement in U.S. Schools." *Educational Researcher* 35 (7): 3–12.

Lamont, Jeffrey H., Cynthia D. Devore, Mandy Allison, Richard Ancona, Stephen E. Barnett, Robert Gunther, Breena Holmes, et al. 2013. "Out-of-School Suspension and Expulsion." *Pediatrics* 131 (3): e1000–1007. https://doi.org/10.1542/peds.2012-3932.

Langley, A. K., A. Gonzalez, C. A. Sugar, D. Solis, and L. Jaycox. 2015. "Bounce Back: Effectiveness of an Elementary School-Based Intervention for Multicultural Children Exposed to Traumatic Events." *Journal of Consulting and Clinical Psychology* 83 (5): 853.

Lee, B. 2016. "Causes and Cures VII: Structural Violence." *Aggression and Violent Behavior* 28: 109–14.

Lee, E., H. Larkin, and N. Esaki. 2017. "Exposure to Community Violence as a New Adverse Childhood Experience Category: Promising Results and Future Considerations." *Families in Society* 98 (1): 69–78. https://doi.org/10.1606/1044-3894.2017.10.

Lee, Meggan J., Clare C. Rittschof, Andrew J. Greenlee, Kedir N. Turi, Sandra L. Rodriguez-Zas, Gene E. Robinson, Steven W. Cole, and Ruby Mendenhall. 2021. "Transcriptomic Analyses of Black Women in Neighborhoods with High Levels of Violence." *Psychoneuroendocrinology* 127 (May): 105174. https://doi.org/10.1016/j.psyneuen.2021.105174.

Lee, T., D. Cornell, A. Gregory, and X. Fan. 2011. "High Suspension Schools and Dropout Rates for Black and White Students." *Education and Treatment of Children* 34 (2): 167–92.

Leflot, G., P. A. C. van Lier, P. Onghena, and H. Colpin. 2013. "The Role of Children's On-Task Behavior in the Prevention of Aggressive Behavior Development and Peer Rejection: A Randomized Controlled Study of the Good Behavior Game in Belgian Elementary Classrooms." *Journal of School Psychology* 51 (2): 187–99. https://doi.org/10.1016/j.jsp.2012.12.006.

Lehrer-Small, A. 2021. "New Data Reveal a 432-Hour In-Person Learning Gap Produced by the Politics of Pandemic Schooling." *The 74*, June 9, 2021. https://www.the74million.org/article/one-fate-two-fates-red-states-blue-states-new-data-reveals-a-432-hour-in-person-learning-gap-produced-by-the-politics-of-pandemic-schooling/.

Lerner, R. M. 2004. *Liberty: Thriving and Civic Engagement among America's Youth*. Thousand Oaks, CA: Sage.

Lerner, R. M., J. B. Almerigi, C. Theokas, and J. V. Lerner. 2005. "Positive Youth Development: A View of the Issues." *Journal of Early Adolescence* 25 (1): 10–16. https://doi.org/10.1177/0272431604273211.

Lerner, J. V., E. P. Bowers, K. Minor, M. J. Boyd, M. K. Mueller, K. L. Schmid, C. M. Napolitano, S. Lewin-Bizan, and R. M. Lerner. 2013. "Positive Youth Development: Processes, Philosophies, and Programs." In *Handbook of Psychology: Developmental Psychology* (2nd ed.), edited by R. M. Lerner, M. A. Easterbrooks, J. Mistry, and I. B. Weiner, 365–92. John Wiley & Sons.

Lesser, Benjamin, M. B. Pell, and Kristina Cooke. 2021. "Special Report: As U.S. Schools Shuttered, Student Mental Health Cratered, Reuters Finds." *Reuters*, March 19, 2021. https://www.reuters.com/article/us-health-coronavirus-students-special-r-idUSKBN2BB16D.

Levin, Benjamin. 2000. "Putting Students at the Centre in Education Reform." *Journal of Educational Change* 1 (2): 155–72. https://doi.org/10.1023/A:1010024225888.

Lewallen, Theresa C., Holly Hunt, William Potts-Datema, Stephanie Zaza, and Wayne Giles. 2015. "The Whole School, Whole Community, Whole Child Model: A New Approach for Improving Educational Attainment and Healthy Development for Students." *Journal of School Health* 85 (11): 729–39. https://doi.org/10.1111/josh.12310.

Lewis-McCoy, L. 2014. *Inequality in the Promised Land: Race, Resources, and Suburban Schooling*. Stanford University Press.

Li, A., M. Harries, and L. F. Ross. 2020. "Re-Opening K–12 Schools in the Era of the Coronavirus Disease 2019: Review of State-level Guidance Addressing Equity Concerns." *Journal of Pediatrics* (227): 38–44. https://doi.org/10.1016/j.jpeds.2020.08.069.

Lindberg, Maya. 2015. "False Sense of Security: Police Make School Safer—Right?" Retrieved from https://www.learningforjustice.org/sites/default/files/general/False%20Sense%20of%20Security%20-%20TT50.pdf.

Lindow, J. C., J. L. Hughes, C. South, L. Gutierrez, E. Bannister, M. H. Trivedi, and M. J. Byerly. 2020. "Feasibility and Acceptability of the Youth Aware of Mental Health (YAM) Intervention in US Adolescents." *Archives of Suicide*

Research: Official Journal of the International Academy for Suicide Research 24 (2): 269–84.

Lindow, J. C., J. L. Hughes, C. South, A. Minhajuddin, L. Gutierrez, E. Bannister, M. H. Trivedi, and M. J. Byerly. 2020. "The Youth Aware of Mental Health Intervention: Impact on Help Seeking, Mental Health Knowledge, and Stigma in U.S. Adolescents." *The Journal of Adolescent Health: Official Publication of the Society for Adolescent Medicine* 67 (1): 101–107.

Lindsay, Constance A., Victoria Lee, and Tracey Lloyd. 2018. "The Prevalence of Police Officers in US Schools." *Urban Institute.* https://www.urban.org/urban-wire/prevalence-police-officers-us-schools.

Lipman, Pauline. 2011. *The New Political Economy of Urban Education: Neoliberalism, Race, and the Right to the City.* Routledge.

Lipscomb, S. T., B. E. Hatfield, H. R. Lewis, and E. Goka-Dubose. 2021. "Effects of Early Adversity on Children in Early Care and Education Programs." *Journal of Applied Science in Southern Africa: JASSA: The Journal of the University of Zimbabwe.*

Liu, J. J., M. Reed, and T. A. Girard. 2017. "Advancing Resilience: An Integrative, Multi-System Model of Resilience." *Personality and Individual Differences* 111: 111–18.

Liu, L. C., and B. R. Flay. 2009. "Evaluating Mediation in Longitudinal Multivariate Data: Mediation Effects for the Aban Aya Youth Project Drug Prevention Program." *Prevention Science* 10 (3): 197–207.

Lofton, R. 2021. "Plessy's Tracks: African American Students Confronting Academic Placement in a Racially Diverse School and African American Community." *Race, Ethnicity and Education.* https://doi.org/10.1080/13613324.2021.1924141.

López, C. M., A. R. Andrews III, A. M. Chisolm, M. A. De Arellano, B. Saunders, and D. Kilpatrick. 2017. "Racial/Ethnic Differences in Trauma Exposure and Mental Health Disorders in Adolescents." *Cultural Diversity and Ethnic Minority Psychology* 23 (3): 382.

Love, H. E., J. Schlitt, S. Soleimanpour, N. Panchal, and C. Behr. 2019. "Twenty Years of School-Based Health Care Growth and Expansion." *Health Affairs* 38 (5): 755–64. https://doi.org/10.1377/hlthaff.2018.05472.

Love, John M., Ellen Eliason Kisker, Christine Ross, Helen Raikes, Jill Constantine, Kimberly Boller, Jeanne Brooks-Gunn, et al. 2005. "The Effectiveness of Early Head Start for 3-Year-Old Children and Their Parents: Lessons for Policy and Programs." *Developmental Psychology* 41 (6): 885–901. https://doi.org/10.1037/0012–1649.41.6.88.

Lundstrum, K. 2018. "Nearly 90 Texas Children Died in Day Care Over the Last Decade, Statesman Reports." *Texas Tribune*, December 6, 2018. https://www.texastribune.org/2018/12/06/texas-day-care-child-deaths-sexual-abuse/.

Lustick, Hilary. 2017. "'Restorative Justice' or Restoring Order? Restorative School Discipline Practices in Urban Public Schools." *Urban Education* 56 (8): 1–28. https://doi.org/10.1177/0042085917741725.

Luthar, S. S., and L. B. Zelazo. 2003. "Research on Resilience: An Integrative Review." *Resilience and Vulnerability: Adaptation in the Context of Childhood Adversities* 2: 510–49.

Lutkus A. D., A. R. Weiss, J. R. Campbell, J. Mazzeo, and S. Lazer. 1999. "The NAEP 1998 Civics Report Card for the Nation" (NCES 2000-457). Institute of Education Sciences, US Department of Education.

Maguire-Jack, Kathryn, Paul Lanier, and Brianna Lombardi. 2020. "Investigating Racial Differences in Clusters of Adverse Childhood Experiences." *American Journal of Orthopsychiatry* 90 (1): 106.

Malka, Adam. 2018. *The Men of Mobtown: Policing Baltimore in the Age of Slavery and Emancipation*. University of North Carolina Press. https://uncpress.org/book/9781469636290/the-men-of-mobtown/.

Mallett, Christopher A. 2016. "The School-to-Prison Pipeline: A Critical Review of the Punitive Paradigm Shift." *Child & Adolescent Social Work Journal* 33 (1): 15–24. https://doi.org/10.1007/s10560-015-0397-1.

Mallett, Christopher A. 2017. "The School-to-Prison Pipeline: Disproportionate Impact on Vulnerable Children and Adolescents." *Education and Urban Society* 49 (6): 563–92. https://doi.org/10.1177/0013124516644053.

Mallett, Christopher A. 2020. "School Shootings and Security Lockdowns: Myths, Positive School Climates, and Safer Campuses." *Juvenile & Family Court Journal* 71 (4): 5–21. https://doi.org/10.1111/jfcj.12184.

Mann, Horace. 1952. "Horace Mann: Eleventh Annual Report Covering the Year 1847." National Education Association. https://genius.com/Horace-mann

-twelfth-annual-report-to-the-secretary-of-the-massachusetts-state-board-of-education-1848-annotated.

Mann, J. J., C. A. Michel, and R. P. Auerbach. 2021. "Improving Suicide Prevention through Evidence-Based Strategies: A Systematic Review." *American Journal of Psychiatry* 178 (7): 611–24. https://doi.org/10.1176/appi.ajp.2020.20060864.

Marcucci, O. 2020. "From the 'Discipline Gap' to 'Hyper-Disciplining': A Discursive Shift in How We Talk about the Disciplining of Black Students." *Teachers College Record.*

Massey, D. S. 1996. "The Age of Extremes: Concentrated Affluence and Poverty in the Twenty-First Century." *Demography* 33 (4): 395–412; discussion 413–16. https://doi.org/10.2307/2061773.

Matos, Alejandra. 2017. "In Missouri, Students Who Bully Could be Charged with a Felony." *Washington Post*, January 6, 2017. https://www.washingtonpost.com/local/education/in-missouri-students-who-bully-could-be-charged-with-a-felony/2017/01/06/0e71f17e-d1e2-11e6-945a-76f69a399dd5_story.html.

McCluskey, G., G. Lloyd, J. Kane, S. Riddell, J. Stead, and E. Weedon. 2008. "Can Restorative Practices in Schools Make a Difference?" *Educational Review* 60 (4): 405–17.

McCoy, D. C., H. Yoshikawa, K. M. Ziol-Guest, G. J. Duncan, H. S. Schindler, K. Magnuson, R. Yang, A. Koepp, and J. P. Shonkoff. 2017. "Impacts of Early Childhood Education on Medium- and Long-Term Educational Outcomes." *Educational Researcher* 46 (8): 474–87. https://doi.org/10.3102/0013189X17737739.

McGee, Ebony O., Portia K. Botchway, Dara E. Naphan-Kingery, Amanda J. Brockman, Stacey Houston, and Devin T. White. 2021. "Racism Camouflaged as Impostorism and the Impact on Black STEM Doctoral Students." *Race Ethnicity and Education* 25 (4): 487–507. https://doi.org/10.1080/13613324.2021.1924137.

McKenna, Joseph M., Kathy Martinez-Prather, and Scott W. Bowman. 2016. "The Roles of School-Based Law Enforcement Officers and How These Roles Are Established: A Qualitative Study." *Criminal Justice Policy Review* 27 (4): 420–43. https://doi.org/10.1177/0887403414551001.

McKenna, Joseph M., and Joycelyn M. Pollock. 2014. "Law Enforcement Officers in Schools: An Analysis of Ethical Issues." *Criminal Justice Ethics* 33 (3): 163–84. https://doi.org/10.1080/0731129X.2014.982974.

McLean, C., L. J. E. Austin, M. Whitebook, and K. L. Olson. 2021. *Early Childhood Workforce Index—2020*. Berkeley, CA: Center for the Study of Child Care Employment, University of California Berkeley. https://cscce.berkeley.edu/workforce-index-2020/report-pdf/.

McLoughlin, G. M., J. A. McCarthy, J. T. McGuirt, C. R. Singleton, C. G. Dunn, and P. Gadhoke. 2020. "Addressing Food Insecurity through a Health Equity Lens: A Case Study of Large Urban School Districts During the COVID-19 Pandemic." *Journal of Urban Health* 97 (6): 759–775. https://doi.org/10.1007/s11524-020-00476-0.

Mendelson, T., S. D. Tandon, L. O'Brennan, P. J. Leaf, and N. S. Ialongo. 2015. "Brief Report: Moving Prevention into Schools: The Impact of a Trauma-Informed School-Based Intervention." *Journal of Adolescence* 43, 142–47.

Menting, B., P. A. C. van Lier, H. M. Koot, D. Pardini, and R. Loeber. 2016. "Cognitive Impulsivity and the Development of Delinquency from Late Childhood to Early Adulthood: Moderating Effects of Parenting Behavior and Peer Relationships." *Development and Psychopathology* 28 (1): 167–83. https://doi.org/10.1017/S095457941500036X.

Merikangas, K. R., J. He, M. Burstein, S. A. Swanson, S. Avenevoli, L. Cui, C. Benjet, K. Georgiades, and J. Swendsen. 2010. "Lifetime Prevalence of Mental Disorders in US Adolescents: Results from the National Comorbidity Study-Adolescent Supplement (NCS-A)." *Journal of the American Academy of Child and Adolescent Psychiatry* 49 (10): 980–89.

Merkwae, Amanda. 2015. "Schooling the Police: Race, Disability, and the Conduct of School Resource Officers." *Michigan Journal of Race and Law* 21 (1): 147–81. https://doi.org/10.36643/mjrl.21.1.schooling.

Merrick, M. T., D. C. Ford, K. A. Ports, A. S. Guinn, J. Chen, J. Klevens, M. Metzler, C. M. Jones, T. R. Simon, V. M. Daniel, P. Ottley, and J. A. Mercy. 2019. "Vital Signs: Estimated Proportion of Adult Health Problems Attributable to Adverse Childhood Experiences and Implications for Prevention—25 States, 2015–2017." *Morbidity and Mortality Weekly Report* 68 (44): 999–1005. http://dx.doi.org/10.15585/mmwr.mm6844e1.

Miller, H. 2021. "Maryland Eyes COVID Vaccines at School Clinics as Eligibility for Children Approaches." *Baltimore Sun*, October 20, 2021. https://www.baltimoresun.com/coronavirus/bs-md-kids-covid-vaccine-baltimore-county-mass-vaccination-site-20211020-n7yhzy3ewfgltoy7s6ywrnj5k4-story.html.

Miranda-Mendizabal, A., P. Castellví, O. Parés-Badell, I. Alayo, J. Almenara, I. Alonso, M. J. Blasco, A. Cebrià, A. Gabilondo, M. Gili, C. Lagares, J. A. Piqueras, T. Rodríguez-Jiménez, J. Rodríguez-Marín, M. Roca, V. Soto-Sanz, G. Vilagut, and J. Alonso. 2019. "Gender Differences in Suicidal Behavior in Adolescents and Young Adults: Systematic Review and Meta-Analysis of Longitudinal Studies." *International Journal of Public Health* 64 (2): 265–283. https://doi.org/10.1007/s00038-018-1196-1.

Mitchell, Anne W. 2005. "Stair Steps to Quality: A Guide for States and Communities Developing Quality Rating Systems for Early Care and Education." United Way of America, Success by 6. http://www.ctearlychildhood.org/uploads/6/3/3/7/6337139/qris_anne_mitchell.pdf.

Mitra, Dana L. 2004. "The Significance of Students: Can Increasing 'Student Voice' in Schools Lead to Gains in Youth Development?" *Teachers College Record* 106 (4): 651–88. https://doi.org/10.1111/j.1467-9620.2004.00354.x.

Mittleman, Joel. 2018a. "A Downward Spiral? Childhood Suspension and the Path to Juvenile Arrest." *Sociology of Education* 91 (3): 183–204. https://doi.org/10.1177/0038040718784603.

Mittleman, Joel. 2018b. "Sexual Orientation and School Discipline: New Evidence from a Population-Based Sample." *Educational Researcher* 47 (3): 181–90.

Mojtabai, R., M. Olfson, and B. Han. 2016. "National Trends in the Prevalence and Treatment of Depression in Adolescents and Young Adults." *Pediatrics* 138 (6): e20161878. https://doi.org/10.1542/peds.2016-1878.

Mongan, P., and R. Walker. 2012. "The Road to Hell Is Paved with Good Intentions: A Historical, Theoretical, and Legal Analysis of Zero-Tolerance Weapons Policies in American Schools." *Preventing School Failure* 56 (4): 232–40.

Moody, Myles. 2016. "From Under-Diagnoses to Over-Representation: Black Children, ADHD, and the School-To-Prison Pipeline." *Journal of African American Studies* 20 (2): 152–63. https://doi.org/10.1007/s12111-016-9325-5.

Moon, R. Y. 2016. "SIDS and Other Sleep-Related Infant Deaths: Evidence Base for 2016 Updated Recommendations for a Safe Infant Sleeping Environment." *Pediatrics* 138 (5) e20162940. https://doi.org/10.1542/peds.2016-2940.

Morgan, A., and E. Ziglio. 2007. "Revitalizing the Evidence Base for Public Health: An Assets Model." *Promotion and Education* 14 (2_suppl), 17–22.

Morgan, Emily, Nina Salomon, Martha Plotkin, and Rebecca Cohen. 2014. *The School Discipline Consensus Report: Strategies from the Field to Keep Students Engaged in School and Out of the Juvenile Justice System.* New York: Council of State Governments Justice Center.

Mowen, Thomas. 2020. "Sociologist Presents Research behind Headlines about School Safety." February 5, 2020. https://bgindependentmedia.org/sociologist-presents-research-behind-headlines-about-school-safety/.

Muschert, Glenn. W., Stuart Henry, Nicole Bracy, and Anthony A. Peguero. 2014. *Responding to School Violence: Confronting the Columbine Effect.* Boulder, CO: Lynne Rienner.

Musci, R. J., S. R. Hart, E. D. Ballard, A. Newcomer, K. Van Eck, N. Ialongo, and H. Wilcox. 2016. "Trajectories of Suicidal Ideation from Sixth through Tenth Grades in Predicting Suicide Attempts in Young Adulthood in an Urban African American Cohort." *Suicide and Life-threatening Behavior* 46 (3): 255–65. https://doi.org/10.1111/sltb.12191.

Musu, Lauren, A. Zhang, K. Wang, J. Zhang, and B. A. Oudekerk. 2019. *Indicators of School Crime and Safety.* Washington, DC: NCES.

Na, Chongmin, and Denise C. Gottfredson. 2013. "Police Officers in Schools: Effects on School Crime and the Processing of Offending Behaviors." *Justice Quarterly: JQ/Academy of Criminal Justice Sciences* 30 (4): 619–50. https://doi.org/10.1080/07418825.2011.615754.

Nance, Jason P. 2016. "Dismantling the School-to-Prison Pipeline: Tools for Change." *Hein Online* 48: 313. https://heinonline.org/hol-cgi-bin/get_pdf.cgi?handle=hein.journals/arzjl48§ion=24.

National Association for the Education of Young Children (NAEYC). 2019. "Defining and Recognizing High-Quality Early Learning Programs: NAEYC's 10 Accreditation Standards." *Teaching Young Children* 13 (1). https://www.naeyc.org/defining-recognizing-high-quality-early-learning-programs.

National Association for the Education of Young Children (NAEYC). 2022. "DAP:

Defining Developmentally Appropriate Practice." https://www.naeyc.org/resources/position-statements/dap/definition.

National Association of Secondary School Principals. 2020. "School Resource Officers and Law Enforcement in Schools." NASSP. June 30, 2020. https://www.nassp.org/school-resource-officers-and-law-enforcement-in-schools/.

National Association of School Resource Officers (NASRO). 2020a. "Basic 40-Hour School Resource Officer Course Outline and Objectives.

National Association of School Resource Officers (NASRO). 2020b. "Frequently Asked Questions." NASRO. https://www.nasro.org/faq/#:~:text=The%20National%20Association%20of%20School,SROs%20that%20NASRO%20has%20trained.

National Center for Education Statistics (NCES). 2018a. "A Closer Look at Charter School Characteristics." Washington, DC: US Department of Education. Retrieved on June 12, 2021, from https://nces.ed.gov/blogs/nces/post/a-closer-look-at-charter-school-characteristics.

National Center for Education Statistics (NCES). 2018b. "Percentage of Persons Age 3 and Over and Ages 3 to 18 with No Internet Access at Home and Percentage Distribution of Those with No Home Access, by Main Reason for Not Having Access and Selected Characteristics: 2010 and 2017" [data set]. US Department of Education. Institute of Education Science, National Center for Education Statistics. https://nces.ed.gov/programs/digest/d18/tables/dt18_702.40.asp.

National Center for Education Statistics (NCES). 2020a. "English Language Learner (ELL) Students Enrolled in Public Elementary and Secondary Schools, by State: Selected Years, Fall 2000 through Fall 2018." US Department of Education. Institute of Education Science, National Center for Education Statistics. https://nces.ed.gov/programs/digest/d20/tables/dt20_204.20.asp?current=yes.

National Center for Education Statistics (NCES). 2020b. "Number and Percentage of Public-School Students Eligible for Free or Reduced-Price Lunch, by State: Selected Years, 2000–01 through 2018–19" [data set]. US Department of Education. Institute of Education Science, National Center for Education Statistics. https://nces.ed.gov/programs/digest/d20/tables/dt20_204.10.asp.

National Center for Education Statistics (NCES). 2020c. "Enrollment in Public

Elementary and Secondary Schools, by Region, State, Jurisdiction: Selected Years, Fall 1990 through Fall 2019" [data set]. US Department of Education. Institute of Education Science, National Center for Education Statistics. https://nces.ed.gov/programs/digest/d20/tables/dt20_203.20.asp.

National Center for Education Statistics (NCES). 2021a. "Public Charter School Enrollment. Condition of Education." US Department of Education, Institute of Education Sciences. https://nces.ed.gov/programs/coe/indicator/cgb.

National Center for Education Statistics (NCES). 2021b. "Children 3 to 21 Years Old Served Under Individuals with Disabilities Education Act (IDEA), Part B, by Type of Disability: Selected Years, 1976–77 through 2019–20" [data set]. US Department of Education. Institute of Education Science, National Center for Education Statistics. https://nces.ed.gov/programs/digest/d20/tables/dt20_204.30.asp.

National Center for Education Statistics (NCES). 2020c. "Enrollment in Public Elementary and Secondary Schools, by Region, State, Jurisdiction: Selected Years, Fall 1990 through Fall 2019" [data set]. US Department of Education. Institute of Education Science, National Center for Education Statistics. https://nces.ed.gov/programs/digest/d20/tables/dt20_203.20.asp.

National Center on Early Childhood Quality Assurance. 2019. Technical Assistance Fact Sheet. Administration for Children and Families. Washington, DC.

National Education Association (NEA). 2020. NEA Position on COVID-19 Vaccines. https://www.nea.org/resource-library/nea-position-covid-19-vaccines.

National Legal Aid and Defender Association. 1973. "National Advisory Commission on Criminal Justice Standards and Goals, the Defense (1973)." https://www.nlada.org/defender-standards/national-advisory-commission.

National Research Council. 2002. *Community Programs to Promote Youth Development*. National Academies Press.

National Survey of Early Care and Education Project Team (NSECEPT). 2016. "Characteristics of Home-Based Early Care and Education Providers: Initial Findings from the National Survey of Early Care and Education." OPRE Report #2016–13. Washington, DC: Office of Planning, Research and Evaluation, Administration for Children and Families, US Department of Health and Human Services.

Newcomer, A. R., K. B. Roth, S. G. Kellam, W. Wang, N. S. Ialongo, S. R. Hart,

B. M. Wagner, and H. C. Wilcox. 2016. "Higher Childhood Peer Reports of Social Preference Mediates the Impact of the Good Behavior Game on Suicide Attempt." *Prevention Science: The Official Journal of the Society for Prevention Research* 17 (2): 145–56. https://doi.org/10.1007/s11121-015-0593-4.

Nguyen, B. M. D., P. Noguera, N. Adkins, and R. T. Teranishi. 2019. "Ethnic Discipline Gap: Unseen Dimensions of Racial Disproportionality in School Discipline." *American Education Research Journal* 56 (5): 1973–2003.

Nock, M. K., J. G. Green, I. Hwang, K. A. McLaughlin, N. A. Sampson, A. M. Zaslavsky, and R. C. Kessler. 2013. "Prevalence, Correlates, and Treatment of Lifetime Suicidal Behavior among Adolescents: Results from the National Comorbidity Survey Replication Adolescent Supplement." *JAMA Psychiatry* 70 (3): 300–10. https://doi.org/10.1001/2013.jamapsychiatry.55.

Noguera, P. A. 2003. "Schools, Prisons, and Social Implications of Punishment: Rethinking Disciplinary Practices." *Theory into Practice* 42 (4): 341–50.

Norman, Marilyn N., and Joy C. Jordani. 2006. "Targeting Life Skills in 4-H." University of Florida. https://edis.ifas.ufl.edu/publication/4H242.

Norris, Floyd. 2009. "Subprime Loans, Corporate-Style, Will Fuel Defaults." *New York Times*, April 24, 2009. https://www.nytimes.com/2009/04/24/business/economy/24norris.html.

Nuzzo, J. B., and J. M. Sharfstein. 2020. "We Have to Focus on Opening Schools, Not Bars." *New York Times*, July 1, 2020. https://www.nytimes.com/2020/07/01/opinion/coronavirus-schools.html.

O'Donnell, L., A. Stueve, D. Wardlaw, and C. O'Donnell. 2003. "Adolescent Suicidality and Adult Support: The Reach for Health Study of Urban Youth." *American Journal of Health Behavior* 27 (6): 633–44. https://doi.org/10.5993/ajhb.27.6.6.

Office for Civil Rights. 2021. *An Overview of Exclusionary Discipline Practices in Public Schools for the 2017–18 School Year.* Washington, DC: US Department of Education.

Office of Head Start. 2023. "History of Head Start." Administration for Children and Families. https://www.acf.hhs.gov/ohs/about/history-head-start.

Office of the Surgeon General. 2021. "The Surgeon General Releases Call to Action to Implement the National Strategy for Suicide Prevention." US Department of Health and Human Services. https://www.hhs.gov/about

/news/2021/01/19/the-surgeon-general-releases-call-to-action-to-implement-the-national-strategy-for-suicide-prevention.html.

Olds, D., J. Eckenrode, C. Henderson, H. Kitzman, J. Powers, R. Cole, K. Sidora, P. Morris, L. Pettitt, and D. Luckey. 1997. "Long-Term Effects of Home Visitation on Maternal Life Course and Child Abuse and Neglect: A 15-Year Follow-Up of a Randomized Trial." *JAMA* 278 (8): 637–43.

O'Leary, C. C., D. A. Frank, W. Grant-Knight, M. Beeghly, M. Augustyn, R. Rose-Jacobs, H. J. Cabral, and K. Gannon. 2006. "Suicidal Ideation among Urban Nine and Ten Year Olds." *Journal of Developmental and Behavioral Pediatrics* 27 (1): 33–39. https://doi.org/10.1097/00004703-200602000-00005.

Orr, Marion. 1999. *Black Social Capital: The Politics of School Reform in Baltimore, 1986–1998*. University Press of Kansas.

Orser, W. Edward. 1994. *Blockbusting in Baltimore: The Edmondson Village Story.* University Press of Kentucky. https://uknowledge.uky.edu/upk_united_states_history/8/.

Overstreet, S., and S. M. Chafouleas. 2016. "Trauma-Informed Schools: Introduction to the Special Issue." *School Mental Health* 8, 1–6.

Owens, Emily G. 2017. "Testing the School-to-Prison Pipeline." *Journal of Policy Analysis and Management: The Journal of the Association for Public Policy Analysis and Management* 36 (1): 11–37. https://doi.org/10.1002/pam.21954.

Paccione-Dyszlewski, M. R. 2016. "Trauma-Informed Schools: A Must." *The Brown University Child and Adolescent Behavior Letter* 32 (7): 8.

Pancer, S. Mark, Linda Rose-Krasnor, and Lisa D. Loiselle. 2002. "Youth Conferences as a Context for Engagement." *New Directions for Youth Development* 96 (Winter): 47–64. https://doi.org/10.1002/yd.26.

Parsons, T. 1937. *The Structure of Social Action*. New York: McGraw-Hill.

Pennell, J. 2006. "Restorative Practices and Child Welfare: Toward an Inclusive Civil Society." *Journal of Social Issues* 62 (2): 259.

Pentek, Christen, and Marla E. Eisenberg. 2018. "School Resource Officers, Safety, and Discipline: Perceptions and Experiences across Racial/Ethnic Groups in Minnesota Secondary Schools." *Children and Youth Services Review* 88 (May): 141–48. https://doi.org/10.1016/j.childyouth.2018.03.008.

Pepler, D. J., and K. L. Bierman. 2018. "With a Little Help from My Friends: The

Importance of Peer Relationships for Social-Emotional Development." University Park, PA: Edna Bennett Pierce Prevention Research Center, The Pennsylvania State University.

Perez, J. 2020, July 28. "Teachers Union Threatens 'Safety Strikes' before Biden Speech." *Politico.* https://www.politico.com/news/2020/07/28/aft-strikes-school-reopening-384133.

Perez, Zeke, and Ben Erwin. 2020. "A Turning Point: School Resource Officers and State Policy." Education Commission of the States.

Perkins, D. F., and G. G. Noam. 2007. "Characteristics of Sports-Based Youth Development Programs." *New Directions for Youth Development* (115): 75–84.

Perry, B. L., and E. W. Morris. 2014. "Suspending Progress: Collateral Consequences of Exclusionary Punishment in Public Schools." *American Sociological Review* 79 (6): 1067–87.

Petras, H., S. G. Kellam, C. H. Brown, B. O. Muthén, N. S. Ialongo, and J. M. Poduska. 2008. "Developmental Epidemiological Courses Leading to Antisocial Personality Disorder and Violent and Criminal Behavior: Effects by Young Adulthood of a Universal Preventive Intervention in First-and Second-Grade Classrooms." *Drug and Alcohol Dependence* 95, S45–S59.

Petras, H., K. E. Masyn, J. A. Buckley, N. S. Ialongo, and S. Kellam. 2011. "Who Is Most at Risk for School Removal? A Multilevel Discrete-Time Survival Analysis of Individual- and Context-Level Influences." *Journal of Educational Psychology* 103 (1), 223–37. https://doi.org/10.1037/a0021545.

Pfeffer, C. R., L. Normandin, and T. Kakuma. 1998. "Suicidal Children Grow Up: Relations Between Family Psychopathology and Adolescents' Lifetime Suicidal Behavior." *Journal of Nervous and Mental Disease* 186 (5): 269–75. https://doi.org/10.1097/00005053-199805000-00002.

Pietila, Antero. 2010. *Not in My Neighborhood: How Bigotry Shaped a Great American City.* Chicago: Ivan R. Dee.

Pilkauskas, N. V., M. Amorim, and R. E. Dunifon. 2020. "Historical Trends in Children Living in Multigenerational Households in the United States: 1870–2018." *Demography* 57, 2269–96. https://doi.org/10.1007/s13524-020-00920-5.

Pittman, K. J., M. Irby, J. Tolman, N. Yohalem, and T. Ferber. 2003. "Preventing

Problems, Promoting Development, Encouraging Engagement: Competing Priorities or Inseparable Goals?" *Forum for Youth Investment*. http://forumfyi.org/node/105.

Policing Project. 2019. "It's Time to Start Collecting Stop Data: A Case for Comprehensive Statewide Legislation." The Policing Project. September 30, 2019. https://www.policingproject.org/news-main/2019/9/27/its-time-to-start-collecting-stop-data-a-case-for-comprehensive-statewide-legislation.

Powell, Michael. 2009. "Bank Accused of Pushing Mortgage Deals on Blacks." *New York Times*, June 7, 2009. https://www.nytimes.com/2009/06/07/us/07baltimore.html.

Power, Garrett. 1983. "Apartheid Baltimore Style: The Residential Segregation Ordinances of 1910–1913." *Maryland Law Review* 42: 289. https://heinonline.org/hol-cgi-bin/get_pdf.cgi?handle=hein.journals/mllr42§ion=16.

Pranis, K. 2005. *The Little Book of Circle Processes: A New/Old Approach to Peacemaking*. Good Books.

Price, Peter. 2008. "When Is a Police Officer an Officer of the Law: The Status of Police Officers in Schools." *Journal of Criminal Law and Criminology* 99, 541.

"QRIS Data Compendium." 2022. Quality Compendium Resources. https://qualitycompendium.org/resources/qriscompendium.org.

Raymond, Barbara. 2010. "Assigning Police Officers to Schools." ASU Center for≈Problem-Oriented Policing. March 1, 2010. https://popcenter.asu.edu/content/assigning-police-officers-schools-0.

Reidman, David, and Desmond O'Neill. 2019. "School Resource Officers." NSSPA. 2019. https://doi.org/10.1007/978-1-4614-5690-2_100642.

Reimer, K. E. 2018. *Adult Intentions, Student Perceptions: How Restorative Justice Is Used in Schools to Control and Engage*. Charlotte, NC: Information Age Publishing.

Reynolds, A. J., J. A. Temple, D. L. Robertson, and E. A. Mann. 2001. "Long-Term Effects of an Early Childhood Intervention on Educational Achievement and Juvenile Arrest: A 15-Year Follow-Up of Low-Income Children in Public Schools." *JAMA: The Journal of the American Medical Association* 285 (18): 2339–46. https://doi.org/10.1001/jama.285.18.2339.

Reynolds, Arthur J., Judy A. Temple, Suh-Ruu Ou, Dylan L. Robertson, Joshua P. Mersky, James W. Topitzes, and Michael D. Niles. 2007. "Effects of a School-

Based, Early Childhood Intervention on Adult Health and Well-Being: A 19-Year Follow-Up of Low-Income Families." *Archives of Pediatrics & Adolescent Medicine* 161 (8): 730–39. https://doi.org/10.1001/archpedi.161.8.730. PMID: 17679653.

Rist, R. 1970. "Student Social Class and Teacher Expectations: The Self-Fulfilling Prophecy in Ghetto Education." *Harvard Educational Review* 40: 411–51.

Rivera-Calderón, Noelia. 2017. "Arrested at the Schoolhouse Gate: Criminal School Disturbance Laws and Children's Rights in Schools." *National Lawyers Guild.* NLG Review. 2017. https://www.nlg.org/nlg-review/article/arrested-at-the-schoolhouse-gate-criminal-school-disturbance-laws-and-childrens-rights-in-schools/.

Robinson, Jo, Georgina Cox, Aisling Malone, Michelle Williamson, Gabriel Baldwin, Karen Fletcher, and Matt O'Brien. 2013. "A Systematic Review of School-Based Interventions Aimed at Preventing, Treating, and Responding to Suicide-Related Behavior in Young People." *Crisis* 34 (3): 164–82. https://doi.org/10.1027/0227-5910/a000168.

Ropek, Lucas. 2019. "Facial Recognition Software on the Rise in U.S. Schools." *Government Tech*. September 26, 2019. http://www.govtech.com/products/facial-recognition-software-on-the-rise-in-us-schools.html.

Rosiak, John. 2009. "Developing Safe Schools Partnerships with Law Enforcement." *Forum on Public Policy* 2009 (1). http://files.eric.ed.gov/fulltext/EJ864815.pdf.

Rosiak, John. 2018. "5 Things to Consider before Posting Cops in Schools." *Dispatch* 11 (2). https://cops.usdoj.gov/html/dispatch/02–2018/cops_in_schools.html.

ross, kihana miraya. 2020. "Opinion." *New York Times*, June 4, 2020. https://www.nytimes.com/2020/06/04/opinion/george-floyd-anti-blackness.html.

Roth, Jodie L., and Jeanne Brooks-Gunn. 2003. "What Is a Youth Development Program? Identification and Defining Principles." In *Enhancing the Life Chances of Youth and Families: Public Service Systems and Public Policy Perspectives vol. 2, Handbook of Applied Developmental Science: Promoting Positive Child, Adolescent, and Family Development through Research, Policies, and Programs*, edited by F. Jacobs, D. Wertlieb, and R. M. Lerner, 197–223. Thousand Oaks, CA: Sage.

Rothstein, R. 2015. "From Ferguson to Baltimore: The Fruits of Government-

Sponsored Segregation." *Journal of Affordable Housing and Community Development Law* 24 (2): 205–10. https://www.jstor.org/stable/26408163.

Rothstein, R., and R. P. Olympia. 2020. "School Nurses on the Front Lines of Healthcare: The Approach to Maintaining Student Health and Wellness during COVID-19 School Closures." *NASN School Nurse* 35 (5): 269–75. https://doi.org/10.1177/1942602X20935612.

Ryan, Joseph B., Antonis Katsiyannis, Jennifer M. Counts, and Jill C. Shelnut. 2018. "The Growing Concerns Regarding School Resource Officers." *Intervention in School and Clinic* 53 (3): 188–92. https://doi.org/10.1177/1053451217702108.

Rylko-Bauer, B., and P. Farmer. 2016. "Structural Violence, Poverty, and Social Suffering." In *The Oxford Handbook of Social Science of Poverty*, edited by D. Brady and L. M. Burton, 47–74. Oxford Press.

Sama-Miller, Emily, Lauren Akers, Andrea Mraz-Esposito, Rebecca Coughlin, and Marykate Zukiewicz. 2017. "Home Visiting Evidence of Effectiveness Review: Executive Summary." https://EconPapers.repec.org/RePEc:mpr:mprres:ab92c1547bc142a6815d64f332358eb3.

Sampson, Robert J., William Julius Wilson, and Hanna Katz. 2018. "Reassessing Toward a Theory of Race, Crime, and Urban Inequality: Enduring and New Challenges in 21st Century America." *Du Bois Review: Social Science Research on Race* 15 (1): 13–34. https://doi.org/10.1017/S1742058X18000140.

Samuels, Christina A. 2022. "We Struggle to Measure Quality Child Care—and Even More to Fund It." The Hechinger Report, February 3, 2022. https://hechingerreport.org/we-struggle-to-measure-quality-child-care-and-even-more-to-fund-it/.

Santiago, C. D., T. Raviv, A. M. Ros, S. K. Brewer, L. M. Distel, S. A. Torres, A. K. Fuller, et al. 2018. "Implementing the Bounce Back Trauma Intervention in Urban Elementary Schools: A Real-World Replication Trial." *School Psychology Quarterly* 33 (1): 1.

Sapiro, Beth, and Alison Ward. 2019. "Marginalized Youth, Mental Health, and Connection with Others: A Review of the Literature." *Child and Adolescent Social Work Journal* 37 (4): 343–57. https://doi.org/10.1007/s10560-019-00628-5.

Schiff, Mara. 2018. "Can Restorative Justice Disrupt the 'School-to-Prison

Pipeline?'" *Contemporary Justice Review* 21 (2): 121–39. https://doi.org/10.1080/10282580.2018.1455509.

Schrade, B. 2013. "Child-Care Deaths Down Sharply in Minnesota." *Star Tribune*, April 4, 2013. https://www.startribune.com/fewer-children-dying-in-minnesota-day-cares/201306931/?refresh=true.

Segawa, E., J. E. Ngwe, Y. Li, B. R. Flay, and Aban Aya Coinvestigators. 2005. "Evaluation of the Effects of the Aban Aya Youth Project in Reducing Violence Among African American Adolescent Males Using Latent Class Growth Mixture Modeling Techniques." *Evaluation Review* 29 (2): 128–48.

Sellman, E., H. Cremin, and G. McCluskey. 2013. *Restorative Approaches to Conflict in Schools: Interdisciplinary Perspectives on Whole School Approaches to Managing Relationships*. London, UK: Routledge. https://doi.org/10.4324/9781315889696.

Sergi, K., A. Coley, and L. Morse. 2017. "Assessing Quality: Rating Systems for Early Childhood Care Centers." Mississippi State University. https://www.researchgate.net/profile/KaterinaSergi/publication/327039835_Symposium_Session_Early_Childhood_Care_Center_Practices_and_Policies_for_High_Quality_Care_and_Learning/links/5c54500c458515a4c7500e0a/Symposium-Session-Early-Childhood-Care-Center-Practices-and-Policies-for-High-Quality-Care-and-Learning.pdf.

Sharfstein, Joshua M., and Christopher C. Morphew. 2020. "The Urgency and Challenge of Opening K-12 Schools in the Fall of 2020." *JAMA* 324 (2): 133–34. https://doi.org/10.1001/jama.2020.10175.

Sharkey, Patrick. 2013. *Stuck in Place: Urban Neighborhoods and the End of Progress Toward Racial Equality*. University of Chicago Press.

Sharkey, Patrick, and Felix Elwert. 2011. "The Legacy of Disadvantage: Multigenerational Neighborhood Effects on Cognitive Ability." *AJS: American Journal of Sociology* 116 (6): 1934–81. https://doi.org/10.1086/660009.

Shedd, C. 2015. *Unequal City: Race, Schools, and Perceptions of Injustice*. New York: Russell Sage Foundation.

Sheftall, A. H., L. Asti, L. M. Horowitz, A. Felts, C. A. Fontanella, J. V. Campo, and J. A. Bridge. 2016. "Suicide in Elementary School-Aged Children and Early Adolescents." *Pediatrics* 138 (4): e20160436. https://doi.org/10.1542/peds.2016-0436.

Sherrod, Lonnie R. 2005. "Ensuring Liberty by Promoting Youth Development." *Human Development* 48 (6): 376–81. https://www.jstor.org/stable/26763859.

Shiller, Jessica, and BMORE Caucus. 2019. "Winning in Baltimore: The Story of How BMORE Put Racial Equity at the Center of Teacher Union Organizing." *Berkeley Review of Education* 9 (1). https://doi.org/10.5070/B89146427.

Shonkoff, Jack P., Linda Richter, Jacques van der Gaag, and Zulfiqar A. Bhutta. 2012. "An Integrated Scientific Framework for Child Survival and Early Childhood Development." *Pediatrics* 129 (2): e460–72. https://doi.org/10.1542/peds.2011-0366.

Singh, A. A., and C. F. Salazar. 2010. "The Roots of Social Justice in Group Work." *The Journal for Specialists in Group Work* 35 (2): 97–104.

Skiba, R. J., C. Chung, M. Trachok, T. L. Baker, A. Sheya, and R. Hughes. 2014. "Parsing Discipline Disproportionality: Contributions of Infraction, Student, and School Characteristics to Out-of-School Suspension and Expulsion." *American Education Research Journal* 51 (4): 640–70.

Skiba, R. J., R. H. Horner, C. G. Chung, M. K. Rausch, S. L. May, and T. Tobin. 2011. "Race Is Not Neutral: A National Investigation of African American and Latino Disproportionality in School Discipline." *School Psychology Review* 40 (1): 85–107.

Skiba, Russell J., Robert S. Michael, Abra Carroll Nardo, and Reece L. Peterson. 2002. "The Color of Discipline: Sources of Racial and Gender Disproportionality in School Punishment." *The Urban Review* 34 (4): 317–42. https://doi.org/10.1023/A:1021320817372.

Skiba, Russell J., and Karega M. Rausch. 2006. "Zero Tolerance, Suspension, and Expulsion: Questions of Equity and Effectiveness." In *Handbook of Classroom Management: Research, Practice, and Contemporary Issues*, edited by C. M. Evertson and C. S. Weinstein, 1063–89. Mahwah, NJ: Erlbaum.

Slopen, N., J. P. Shonkoff, M. A. Albert, H. Yoshikawa, A. Jacobs, R. Stoltz, and D. Williams. 2016. "Racial Disparities in Child Adversity in the US: Interactions with Family Immigration History and Income." *American Journal of Preventive Medicine* 50 (1): 47–56.

Smerdon, Becky, and Jennifer Cohen. 2009. "Evaluation Findings from High School Reform Efforts in Baltimore." *Journal of Education for Students Placed at Risk* (JESPAR) 14 (3): 238–55. https://doi.org/10.1080/10824660903375693.

Soole, R., K. Kõlves, and D. De Leo. 2015. "Suicide in Children: A Systematic Review." *Archives of Suicide: Official Journal of the International Academy for Suicide Research* 19 (3) 285–304. https://doi.org/10.1080/13811118.2014.996694.

Soto, I. 2020. "Childcare and Returning to Work." American Action Forum, Insight. https://www.americanactionforum.org/insight/childcare-and-returning-to-work/.

Sprague, J. R., C. G. Vincent, T. J. Tobin, and M. Pavid. 2013. "Preventing Disciplinary Exclusions of Students from American Indian/Alaska Native Backgrounds." *Family Court Review* 51 (3): 452–59.

Stein, B. D., L. H. Jaycox, S. H. Kataoka, M. Wong, W. Tu, M. N. Elliott, and A. Fink. 2003. "A Mental Health Intervention for Schoolchildren Exposed to Violence: A Randomized Controlled Trial. *JAMA* 290 (5): 603–11.

Stone, D. M., K. M. Holland, B. Bartholow, A. E. Crosby, S. Davis, and N. Wilkins. 2017. "Preventing Suicide: A Technical Package of Policies, Programs, and Practices." Atlanta, GA: National Center for Injury Prevention and Control, Centers for Disease Control and Prevention.

Stovall, D. 2020. "On Knowing: Willingness, Fugitivity and Abolition in Precarious Times." *Journal of Language and Literacy Education* 16 (1): 1–7.

Strauss, V. 2020, May 25. "Trump Tweets Schools Should Open 'ASAP' (after a Fox News Host Said the Same Thing Sunday Night). Here Are Some Responses." *Washington Post*. https://www.washingtonpost.com/education/2020/05/25/trump-tweets-schools-should-open-asap-after-fox-news-host-said-same-thing-sunday-night-here-are-some-responses/.

Stringfield, Samuel C., and Mary E. Yakimowski-Srebnick. 2005. "Promise, Progress, Problems, and Paradoxes of Three Phases of Accountability: A Longitudinal Case Study of the Baltimore City Public Schools." *American Educational Research Journal* 42 (1): 43–75. http://www.jstor.org/stable/3699455.

Strompolis, M., W. Tucker, E. Crouch, and E. Radcliff. 2019. "The Intersectionality of Adverse Childhood Experiences, Race/Ethnicity, and Income: Implications for Policy." *Journal of Prevention and Intervention in the Community* 47 (4): 310–324.

Stubenbort, Karen, Meredith M. Cohen, and Veronica Trybalski. 2010. "The Effectiveness of an Attachment-Focused Treatment Model in a Therapeutic

Preschool for Abused Children." *Clinical Social Work Journal* 38 (1): 51–60. https://doi.org/10.1007/s10615-007-0107-3.

Substance Abuse and Mental Health Services Administration (SAMHSA). 2012. "SAMHSA's Concept of Trauma and Guidance for a Trauma-Informed Approach." SAMHSA. https://store.samhsa.gov/product/SAMHSA-s-Concept-of-Trauma-and-Guidance-for-a-Trauma-Informed-Approach/SMA14–4884.

Substance Abuse and Mental Health Services Administration (SAMHSA). 2014. "SAMHSA's Concept of Trauma and Guidance for a Trauma-Informed Approach." SAMHSA. https://www.samhsa.gov/resource/dbhis/samhsas-concept-trauma-guidance-trauma-informed-approach.

Substance Abuse and Mental Health Services Administration (SAMHSA). 2018. "Key Substance Use and Mental Health Indicators in the United States: Results from the 2017 National Survey on Drug Use and Health" (HHS Publication No. SMA 18–5068, NSDUH Series H-53).

Thompson, R., E. Briggs, D. J. English, H. Dubowitz, L. C. Lee, K. Brody, M. D. Everson, and W. M. Hunter. 2005. "Suicidal Ideation among 8-Year-Olds Who Are Maltreated and at Risk: Findings from the LONGSCAN Studies." *Child Maltreatment* 10 (1): 26–36. https://doi.org/10.1177/1077559504271271.

Thorsborne, M., and P. Blood. 2013. *Implementing Restorative Practices in Schools: A Practical Guide to Transforming School Communities.* Jessica Kingsley Publishers.

Thurau, Lisa H., and Johanna Wald. 2009. "Controlling Partners: When Law Enforcement Meets Discipline in Public Schools." HEIN Online. 54: 977. https://heinonline.org/hol-cgi-bin/get_pdf.cgi?handle=hein.journals/nyls54§ion=51.

Todres, J., and L. Meeler. 2021. "Confronting Housing Insecurity—A Key to Getting Kids Back to School." *JAMA Pediatrics* 175 (9): 889–90.

Tomek, S., L. M. Hooper, W. T. Church II, K. A. Bolland, J. M. Bolland, and K. Wilcox. 2015. "Relations among Suicidality, Recent/Frequent Alcohol Use, and Gender in a Black American Adolescent Sample: A Longitudinal Investigation." *Journal of Clinical Psychology* 71 (6): 544–60. https://doi.org/10.1002/jclp.22169.

Tout, Kathryn, Katherine Magnuson, Shannon Lipscomb, Lynn Karoly, Rebecca Starr, Heather Quick, Diane Early, Dale Epstein, Gail Joseph, Kelly Maxwell,

Joanne Roberts, Christopher Swanson, and Jennifer Wenner. 2017. *Validation of the Quality Ratings Used in Quality Rating and Improvement Systems (QRIS): A Synthesis of State Studies*. OPRE Report #2017–92. Washington, DC: Office of Planning, Research and Evaluation, Administration for Children and Families, US Department of Health and Human Services.

Twum-Antwi, A., P. Jefferies, and M. Ungar. 2020. "Promoting Child and Youth Resilience by Strengthening Home and School Environments: A Literature Review." *International Journal of School and Educational Psychology* 8 (2): 78–89.

Ullrich, R., S. Schmit, and R. Cosse. 2019. "Inequitable Access to Childcare Subsidies." Center for Law and Social Policy, Washington, DC. https://www.clasp.org/publications/report/brief/inequitable-access-child-care-subsidies.

Ungar, M. 2011. *The Social Ecology of Resilience: A Handbook of Theory and Practice*. Springer Science & Business Media.

United States Commission on Civil Rights. 2019. "Beyond Suspensions: Examining School Discipline Policies and Connections to the School-to-Prison Pipeline for Students of Color with Disabilities." https://www.usccr.gov/reports/2019/beyond-suspensions-examining-school-discipline-policies-and-connections-school-prison.

United States Congress. 1993. Gun-Free Schools Act of 1993–1994. http://www.congress.gov/.

United Nations Human Rights. 2016. "Statement to the Media by the United Nations' Working Group of Experts on People of African Descent, on the Conclusion of Its Official Visit to USA, 19–29 January 2016." Office of the High Commissioner. 2016. http://www.ohchr.org/EN/NewsEvents/Pages/DisplayNews.aspx?NewsID=17000&LangID=E.

US Department of Education. 2016. "Civil Rights Data Collection." Retrieved August 1, 2021, from https://ocrdata.ed.gov/.

US Department of Education. 2021a. "Education in a Pandemic: The Disparate Impacts of COVID-19 on America's Students." https://www2.ed.gov/about/offices/list/ocr/docs/20210608-impacts-of-covid19.pdf.

US Department of Education. 2021b. Civil Rights Data Collection. https://ocrdata.ed.gov/.

US Department of Health and Human Services and the Office of the Surgeon General. 2021. "The Surgeon General's Call to Action to Implement the

National Strategy for Suicide Prevention." US Department of Health & Human Services.

US Department of Health and Human Services and US Department of Education. 2023. "Policy Statement of Inclusion of Children with Disabilities in Early Education Programs." Washington, DC. https://sites.ed.gov/idea/files/policy-statement-on-inclusion-11-28-2023.pdf.

US Department of Justice (DOJ). 2021. "Department of Justice Awards More Than $125 Million in Grants under the Stop School Violence Act." https://www.justice.gov/usao-ndtx/pr/department-justice-awards-more-125-million-grants-under-stop-school-violence-act.

US Department of Justice (DOJ) and National Association of School Resource Officers (NASRO). 2022. "34 USC 10389: Definitions." 2022. https://uscode.house.gov/view.xhtml?req=(title:34%20section:10389%20edition:prelim).

US Department of Justice (DOJ) and US Department of Education. 2014. "Dear Colleague Letter on the Nondiscriminatory Administration of School Discipline." Retrieved from https://www2.ed.gov/about/offices/list/ocr/letters/colleague-201401-title-vi.html.

US Food and Drug Administration (FDA). 2024. Emergency use authorization. U.S. Food and Drug Administration. https://www.fda.gov/emergency-preparedness-and-response/mcm-legal-regulatory-and-policy-framework/emergency-use-authorization#vaccines.

Vaandering, D. 2010. "The Significance of Critical Theory for Restorative Justice in Education." *Review of Education, Pedagogy, and Cultural Studies* 32 (2): 145–76. https://doi.org/10.1080/10714411003799165

Valdez, Avelardo, Charles D. Kaplan, and Russell L. Curtis Jr. 2007. "Aggressive Crime, Alcohol and Drug Use, and Concentrated Poverty in 24 U.S. Urban Areas." *American Journal of Drug and Alcohol Abuse* 33 (4): 595–603. https://doi.org/10.1080/00952990701407637.

Van Breda, A. D. 2001. "Resilience Theory: A Literature Review." Pretoria, South Africa: *South African Military Health Service.*

van der Kolk, Bessel A., Susan Roth, David Pelcovitz, Susanne Sunday, and Joseph Spinazzola. 2005. "Disorders of Extreme Stress: The Empirical Foundation of a Complex Adaptation to Trauma." *Journal of Traumatic Stress* 18 (5): 389–99. https://doi.org/10.1002/jts.20047.

van Lier, Pol A. C., Patricia Vuijk, and Alfons. A. M. Crijnen. 2005. "Understanding Mechanisms of Change in the Development of Antisocial Behavior: The Impact of a Universal Intervention." *Journal of Abnormal Child Psychology* 33 (5): 521–35. https://doi.org/10.1007/s10802-005-6735-7.

Vavrus, F., and Cole, K. 2002. "'I Didn't Do Nothin': The Discursive Construction of School Suspension." *The Urban Review* 34 (2): 87–111.

Virginia Department of Criminal Justice Services. 2021. "School Resource Officer and School Administrator Basic Course." https://www.dcjs.virginia.gov/content/school-resource-officer-and-school-administrator-basic-course-1.

Vision for Baltimore. 2020. Visionforbaltimore.com.

Wachtel, T., and P. McCold. 2001. "Restorative Justice in Everyday Life." In *Restorative Justice and Civil Society*, edited by H. Strang and J. Braithwaite, 114–29. Cambridge University Press.

Wacquant, L. 1997. "The Pernicious Premises in the Study of the American Ghetto." *International Journal of Urban and Regional Research* 21 (2): 341–53. doi.org/10.1111/1468-2427.00076.

Wade, D. T., and K. S. Ortiz. 2017. "Punishing Trauma: How Schools Contribute to the Carceral Continuum through Its Response to Traumatic Experiences." In *Understanding, Dismantling, and Disrupting the Prison-to-School Pipeline*, edited by K. J. Fashing-Varner, L. Martin, R. Mitchell, K. Bennett-Haron, and A. Daneshzadeh, 183–93. Lanham, MD: Lexington Books.

Walker, T. 2021. "Educators Should Receive Priority Access to COVID Vaccine." National Education Association. https://www.nea.org/advocating-for-change/new-from-nea/nea-educators-should-receive-priority-access-covid-vaccine.

Walkley, M., and T. L. Cox. 2013. "Building Trauma-Informed Schools and Communities." *Children and Schools* 35 (2): 123–26.

Wall, C. R. G. 2021. "Relationship Over Reproach: Fostering Resilience by Embracing a Trauma-Informed Approach to Elementary Education." *Journal of Aggression, Maltreatment and Trauma* 30 (1): 118–37.

Wasserman, D., V. Carli, C. Wasserman, A. Apter, J. Balazs, J. Bobes, R. Bracale, et al. 2010. "Saving and Empowering Young Lives in Europe (SEYLE): A Randomized Controlled Trial." *BMC Public Health* 10, 192. https://doi.org/10.1186/1471-2458-10-192.

Wasserman, D., C. W. Hoven, C. Wasserman, M. Wall, R. Eisenberg, G. Hadlaczky, I. Kelleher, et al. 2015. “School-based Suicide Prevention Programs: The SEYLE Cluster-Randomized, Controlled Trial.” *Lancet* (London, England) 385 (9977): 1536–44. https://doi.org/10.1016/S0140-6736(14)61213-7.

Weber, Constanze, and Leen Vereenooghe. 2020. “Reducing Conflicts in School Environments Using Restorative Practices: A Systematic Review.” *International Journal of Educational Research Open* 1 (January): 100009. https://doi.org/10.1016/j.ijedro.2020.100009.

Wechsler, M., H. Melnick, A. Maier, and J. Bishop. 2016. *The Building Blocks of High-Quality Early Childhood Education Programs* (policy brief). Palo Alto, CA: Learning Policy Institute.

Weddle, E. 2014. “Death Toll of Children at Indiana Day Cares Hits 31.” *Indy Star*, March 9, 2014. https://www.indystar.com/story/news/2014/03/09/death-toll-of-children-at-indiana-day-cares-hits-31/6232167/.

Weiler, Spencer C., and Martha Cray. 2011. “Police at School: A Brief History and Current Status of School Resource Officers.” *The Clearing House: A Journal of Educational Strategies, Issues and Ideas* 84 (4): 160–63. https://doi.org/10.1080/00098655.2011.564986.

Weiner, Dana, Leanne Heaton, Mike Stiehl, Brian Chor, Kiljoong Kim, Kurt Heisler, Richard Foltz, and Amber Farrell. 2020. “COVID-19 and Child Welfare: Using Data to Understand Trends in Maltreatment and Response.” Issue Brief. *Chapin Hall at the University of Chicago.*

Weingarten R. 2020, December 20. *New Hope for a New Year.* American Federation of Teachers, AF-CIO. https://www.aft.org/node/18828.

Weisburst, Emily K. 2019. “Patrolling Public Schools: The Impact of Funding for School Police on Student Discipline and Long-Term Education Outcomes.” *Journal of Policy Analysis and Management* 38 (2): 338–65. https://doi.org/10.1002/pam.22116.

Welch, Kelly, and Allison Ann Payne. 2018. “Zero Tolerance School Policies.” In *The Palgrave International Handbook of School Discipline, Surveillance, and Social Control*, edited by Jo Deakin, Emmeline Taylor, and Aaron Kupchik, 215–34. Cham: Springer International Publishing. https://doi.org/10.1007/978-3-319-71559-9_11.

Welsh, Richard O., and Shafiqua Little. 2018. “The School Discipline Dilemma: A Comprehensive Review of Disparities and Alternative Approaches.” *Review of Educational Research* 88 (5): 752–94. https://doi.org/10.3102/0034654318791582.

Whitaker, A., S. Torres-Guillén, M. Morton, H. Jordan, S. Coyle, A. Mann, and W.-L. Sun. 2019. "Cops and No Counselors: How the Lack of School Mental Health Staff Is Harming Students." ACLU. Retrieved August 1, 2021, from https://www.aclu.org/issues/juvenile-justice/school-prison-pipeline/cops-and-no-counselors.

White, A., L. C. Liburd, and F. Coronado. 2021. "Addressing Racial and Ethnic Disparities in COVID-19 among School-Aged Children: Are We Doing Enough?" *Preventing Chronic Disease* 18. https://doi.org/10.5888/pcd18.210084.

The White House. 2021. "Executive Order 14043 of September 9, 2021: Requiring Coronavirus Disease 2019 Vaccination for Federal Employees." Vol. 86, No. 175.

Whitehurst, G. J. 2019. "Why the Federal Government Should Subsidize Childcare and How to Pay for It." *Evidence Speaks Reports* 2 (11), Economic Studies at Brookings. https://www.brookings.edu/articles/why-the-federal-government-should-subsidize-childcare-and-how-to-pay-for-it/.

Wiest-Stevenson, C., and C. Lee. 2016. "Trauma-Informed Schools." *Journal of Evidence-Informed Social Work* 13 (5): 498–503.

Wilcox, H. C., S. G. Kellam, C. H. Brown, J. M. Poduska, N. S. Ialongo, W. Wang, et al. 2008. "The Impact of Two Universal Randomized First-and Second-grade Classroom Interventions on Young Adult Suicide Ideation and Attempts. *Drug and Alcohol Dependence* 95, S60–S73.

Williams, G., and M. Yogman M. 2023. "Addressing Early Education and Child Care Expulsion." *Pediatrics* 123 (5). https://doi.org/10.1542/peds.2023-064049.

Wilson, Scot. 2016. "The Debate over Police Officers in Schools." Close Up Foundation. February 16, 2021. https://closeup.org/the-debate-over-school-resource-officers-and-the-counselorsnotcops-campaign/.

Wilson, W. J. 1987. *The Truly Disadvantaged: The Inner City, the Underclass, and Public Policy.* Chicago: University of Chicago Press.

Wilson, W. J. 1997. *When Work Disappears: The World of the New Urban Poor.* New York: Vintage Books.

Winn, M. T. 2018. *Justice on Both Sides: Transforming Education through Restorative Justice*. Harvard Education Press.

Witvliet, M., P. A. C. van Lier, P. Cuijpers, and H. M. Koot. 2009. "Testing Links between Childhood Positive Peer Relations and Externalizing Outcomes through a Randomized Controlled Intervention Study." *Journal of Consulting and Clinical Psychology* 77 (5): 905–15. https://doi.org/10.1037/a0014597.

Wolf, Kerrin C. 2014. "Arrest Decision Making by School Resource Officers." *Youth Violence and Juvenile Justice* 12 (2): 137–51. https://doi.org/10.1177/1541204013491294.

Wolf, K. C., and A. Kupchik. 2017. "School Suspensions and Adverse Experiences in Adulthood." *Justice Quarterly* 34 (3): 407–30.

Woodworth, Katrina R., Jane L. David, Roneeta Guha, Haiwen Wang, and Alejandro Lopez-Torkos. 2008. "San Francisco Bay Area KIPP Schools: A Study of Early Implementation and Achievement." Final report. Menlo Park, CA: SRI International. http://www.kippbayarea.org/wp-content/uploads/2010/06/SRI-International-Report.pdf.

Workman, S., and S. Jessen-Howard. 2018. "Understanding the True Cost of Childcare for Infants and Toddlers." Center for American Progress, Washington, DC. https://www.americanprogress.org/issues/earlychildhood/reports/2018/11/15/460970/understanding-true-cost-child-care-infants-toddlers/.

World Health Organization. n.d. "Constitution." https://www.who.int/about/accountability/governance/constitution.

Wrigley, Julia, and Joanna Dreby. 2005. "Fatalities and the Organization of Child Care in the United States, 1985–2003." *American Sociological Review* 70 (5): 729–57. https://doi.org/10.1177/000312240507000501.

Yard, Ellen, Lakshmi Radhakrishnan, Michael F. Ballesteros, Michael Sheppard, Abigail Gates, Zachary Stein, Kathleen Hartnett, et al. 2021. "Emergency Department Visits for Suspected Suicide Attempts Among Persons Aged 12–25 Years before and during the COVID-19 Pandemic – United States, January 2019-May 2021." *Morbidity and Mortality Weekly Report* 70 (24): 888–94. https://doi.org/10.15585/mmwr.mm7024e1.

Yildiz, Muhammed, Emirhan Demirhan, and Suheyl Gurbuz. 2019. "Contextual Socioeconomic Disadvantage and Adolescent Suicide Attempts: A Multilevel

Investigation." *Journal of Youth and Adolescence* 48 (4): 802–14. https://doi.org/10.1007/s10964-018-0961-z.

Yohalem, Nicole, Nalini Ravindranath, Karen Pittman, and Danielle Evennou. 2010. "Ready by 21: Insulating the Education Pipeline to Increase Postsecondary Success." Forum for Youth Investments, September 2010. https://www.newenglandssc.org/wp-content/uploads/2015/11/rb21_credentialed-by-26_brief-1_1_.pdf.

Young, Douglas, Christina Yancey, Sara Betsinger, and Jill Farrell. 2011. "Disproportionate Minority Contact in the Maryland Juvenile Justice System." Institute for Governmental Service and Research. University of Maryland, College Park. https://www.ojp.gov/ncjrs/virtual-library/abstracts/disproportionate-minority-contact-maryland-juvenile-justice-system.

Zehr, H. 2015. *The Little Book of Restorative Justice: Revised and Updated.* Simon and Schuster.

Zeldin, Shepherd, Josset Sky Gauley, Alexandra Barringer, and Brie Chapa. 2018. "How High Schools Become Empowering Communities: A Mixed-Method Explanatory Inquiry into Youth-Adult Partnership and School Engagement." *American Journal of Community Psychology* 61 (3–4): 358–71. https://doi.org/10.1002/ajcp.12231.

Zeng, Songtian, Catherine P. Corr, Courtney O'Grady, and Yiyang Guan. 2019. "Adverse Childhood Experiences and Preschool Suspension Expulsion: A Population Study." *Child Abuse and Neglect* 97 (November): 104149. https://doi.org/10.1016/j.chiabu.2019.104149.

Zimmerman, Marc A. 2013. "Resiliency Theory: A Strengths-Based Approach to Research and Practice for Adolescent Health." *Health Education and Behavior: The Official Publication of the Society for Public Health Education* 40 (4): 381–83. https://doi.org/10.1177/1090198113493782.

Zippel, Claire, and Arloc Sherman. 2021. "Bolstering Family Income Is Essential to Helping Children Emerge Successfully from the Current Crisis." *CBPP*, updated February 25, 2021. https://www.cbpp.org/research/poverty-and-inequality/bolstering-family-income-is-essential-to-helping-children-emerge.

Index